THE
PLAGUE
RACE

Also by Edward Marriott

THE LOST TRIBE

WILD SHORE

THE
PLAGUE
RACE

A TALE OF FEAR, SCIENCE AND HEROISM

Edward Marriott

PICADOR

First published 2002 by Picador
an imprint of Pan Macmillan Ltd
Pan Macmillan, 20 New Wharf Road, London N1 9RR
Basingstoke and Oxford
Associated companies throughout the world
www.panmacmillan.com

ISBN 0 330 48318 8

Illustrations on pp. viii and 273 © Institut Pasteur, reproduced by permission.
Drawing of flea by Paul-Louis Simond on p. xi © Institut Pasteur, reproduced by permission.
Illustration on p. ix © The Kitasato Institute, reproduced by permission.

1 3 5 7 9 8 6 4 2

A CIP catalogue record for this book is available from
the British Library.

Typeset by Intype London Ltd
Printed and bound in Great Britain by
Mackays of Chatham plc, Chatham, Kent

for Grandfather

Author's note

This is a work of non-fiction, and the characters and events described are real, with one exception. The story of Mohanlal and Hetal was constructed using the first-hand accounts of many of the refugees from the Surat plague of 1994.

Human destiny is bound to remain a gamble, because at some unpredictable time and in some unforeseeable manner nature will strike back.

Mirage of Health, RENÉ DUBOS, 1959

Cities are the graveyards of mankind.

JOHN CAIRNS, British biochemist

In observation and experiment, chance favours only the prepared mind.

LOUIS PASTEUR

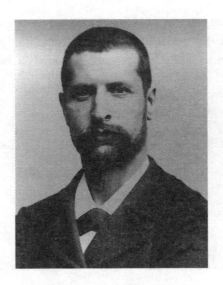

Dr Alexandre Yersin, c. 1894

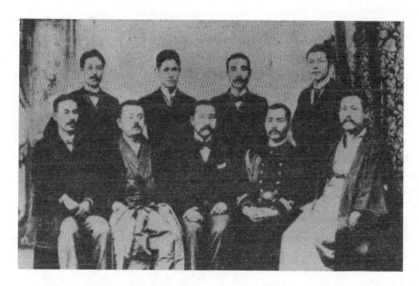

*Professor Shibasaburo (front row, second from left) with colleagues
and assistants, Tokyo 1894, on his return from Hong Kong*

Plague (plāg). **1.** Any disease of wide prevalence or excessive mortality. **2.** An acute infectious disease caused by the bacterium *Yersinia pestis* and marked clinically by high fever, toxemia, prostration, a petechial eruption, lymph node enlargement, and pneumonia, or hemorrhage from the mucous membranes; primarily a disease of rodents, transmitted to humans by fleas that have bitten infected animals.

PDR Medical Dictionary

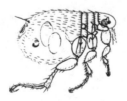

Prologue

LATE ONE AFTERNOON, as the mango and banana sellers were beginning to count their day's takings and the Hong Kong street lights were stuttering into life, a monstrous rat surfaced at the intersection of Aberdeen and Bridges. The size of a small cat, it emerged from the drain on one side of the road and climbed up and out, its fur glistening and matted. The rat moved slowly and heavily, with a corpulent waddle, belly low to the ground, mouth open. It rolled its shoulders as it ran, shifting its weight old-mannishly, as if even this short a distance was hugely effortful. As the animal reached the fruit stall on the other side and lumbered to the pavement, the vendor began screaming. She ran out from behind the clumps of bananas with a broom, stamping her feet till all the other stallkeepers heard her and ran to join in. Then there were six of them yelping curses, thrusting through the fruit boxes with broom handles as the rat, with sublime nonchalance, sniffed along the back edge of the pavement and disappeared into a hole no bigger than a small coin.

*

A CENTURY EARLIER, 1894, the same huddled streets, the same rodents. Bubonic plague, exploding out of southern China, had torn through the island colony and now the houses lay shuttered and boarded-up, the only movement through the narrow alleyways the slow shuffle of soldiers, doctors, scientists. Plague, the most feared and least understood of all contagious diseases, was back; for the researchers gathered in the city, cracking the code was the greatest prize of all.

In Hong Kong, at the start of a global meltdown known today as the third plague pandemic, the competition focused on two scientists: the renowned Japanese bacteriologist Professor Shibasaburo Kitasato and his French counterpart, Dr Alexandre Yersin. For Yersin, whose passion for research had been manifest from childhood, Hong Kong was a crucible, his defining moment. For Kitasato, confident of victory, 1894 would prove an equal crux, though for utterly different reasons.

*

IF EVER THERE WAS a time to be a scientist – and most particularly a bacteriologist – it was as the nineteenth century approached its close. The 1870s and 1880s, the years of Yersin's adolescence and early career, were also the era when epidemic diseases first began to lose their primacy over man – something that must have served both as thrill and inspiration. Science was catching up, learning faster than the diseases could mutate. Leprosy, typhoid fever, malaria, tuberculosis, diphtheria and tetanus – all these were now understood, their causal agents pinned down by the powerful new techniques of bacteriology.

Born in Switzerland, Yersin arrived in Paris in August 1885, when he was almost twenty-two. This was the newly minted, architecturally logical and expansive metropolis of Baron Georges Eugène Haussmann, a place of gleaming broad-swept boulevards and avenues, a magnet for Europe's wealthiest sophisticates. And here was Yersin, struggling to get his suitcases off the train, head down as he beetled for his first appointment, the glinting sunshine on the pale stone of the buildings little more than a distraction from the main business: his transformation from darkly intense scientific amateur to practised and increasingly intuitive medical technician.

His timing was perfect: less than ten days before, on 25 July, Louis Pasteur, pioneering the use of rabies inoculation, had successfully cured his first patient. Over the next five years, Yersin would work at the Pasteur Institute as personal assistant and *préparateur* to Pasteur's colleague Dr Émile Roux in his researches on tuberculosis and diphtheria; win the 1888 Paris Medical Faculty bronze medal for his thesis on tuberculosis; spend two months on Robert Koch's Berlin bacteriology course; and, in 1890, flee to become a ship's doctor in the Far East, a move so sudden and unexpected that even today one hears bacteriologists muttering in sinister tones of 'scandal', certain their hero had committed some shameful act which condemned him, thenceforth, to be always in flight.

It is more likely, though, that he was running from something far less shadowy, that he was embracing adventure as much as escaping the constraints of his upbringing, academic life and the social whirl of Paris. He'd always avoided parties, protesting in letters home at the pretension and vapidity of Paris society, and before long he was engineering excuses to flee: a solitary canoeing trip to the coast, 'sick leave' from which he would return suspiciously tanned and relaxed.

He was a man who preferred solitude to the company

of others, who never had a relationship with a woman, whose only attempt at courtship met with rebuff. Every day he wrote to his mother, and with her at least he was open, happy to express feelings of inadequacy or isolation, as if she alone would not judge.

He never knew his father – a scientist too – who died three weeks before his birth. He was raised by women: his mother, sister, and surrounded from boyhood by the ballooning skirts of the young women who attended his mother's Swiss finishing school. To him the girls were 'apes' as, throughout his life, all females would be. He had a brother, barely a year older, but it is hard to see how the two of them could have come from the same stock: the elder, Franck, was athletic, raucous, sunny; Alexandre was shy, saturnine, interior.

Perhaps the shadow of his mother blighted his relationships with women: her letters feel claustrophobic, with her constant refrain of 'Why don't you marry?' and continual need for reassurance about the path of his career. He grew to covet his own privacy, betraying mounting irritation at the students assigned to him: 'As soon as [they] have gone,' he'd typically complain, 'I will be happy. The laboratory will finally be mine and will be peaceful again.' To his mother – a rigorous, old-school Protestant – he admitted only a single flirtation, and one imagines the candidate was a young woman of whom he was certain she'd approve. Mina Schwartzenbach was a student, the niece of one of his mother's friends. Revealingly, he told his mother of the possibility before even consulting young Mina, explaining that he 'might consider' courting her: the language of youthful arrogance, born of insecurity. And it was this bundle of neuroses that Mina, days later, was quick to reject.

Never again – to family or colleagues – did Yersin express interest in a woman.

Likewise, he spoke of his father to no one – neither schoolfriends, nor his mother, nor his brother. Yet Alexandre Sr. continued to exert power: an invisible weight, driving the son onwards, maybe in his absence creating Yersin's manifest ambition. Psychotherapists have argued that sons deprived of fathers work harder to make their mark – Sartre, who lost his when he was two, claimed the death 'gave me my liberty', thus freeing him for artistic achievement – and so, perhaps, it was with Yersin.

*

To FRIENDS, COLLABORATORS, even long-time colleagues, he was always simply 'Yersin', his first name a mystery until his obituaries in 1943. Through his fierceness, his lifelong self-imposed exile from home, his pride and committed friendships with children, one senses a loneliness that could only be assuaged by work, by immersion in that which felt manageable.

He dressed simply, and can be seen posing stiff-backed, uncertain and unsmiling, in the handful of surviving photographs. He eschewed alcohol, secured his pocket watch to his belt loop with a length of household string, taught himself astronomy and, in old age, grew to love aeroplanes. At the age of eight, in an early display of passion for scientific research, he killed his mother's cat. He secured the noose to a ceiling timber, dragged a table underneath, set out a bowl of chopped steak and enticed the cat onward. While the animal ate he inched the noose under the chin, over the ears, watched the rope cord divide the downy throat fur. Then, before the cat could even look up, the boy hooked his fingers under the table edge and pulled hard. Fifteen minutes later he had it spreadeagled on the bread board, its belly scissored open, spleen and heart sectioned and numbered, swabbing blood, urine and faeces on to microscope slides.

The same year, his sense of destiny forming, he discovered a trunk belonging to his late father wedged behind suitcases in a far corner of the attic at his home at Morges, in Switzerland. The boy as detective, sifting the past, alive to its freight and meaning, found much that was mundane – razors, shoehorns, a balding hairbrush – but also other items that seemed to speak directly to him, that felt perhaps as though his father had planted them there, certain that his son, sooner or later, would come looking. These were the tools of the naturalist's profession, the scalpels and callipers and microscopes his father used in his studies of insects. To the boy, turning them over and over in his hands, testing their mechanism and examining the manufacturers' stamps under the dim attic bulb, they must have felt smooth, quickly warm, as if they'd not long left his father's hands.

But it was in adventure that the adult Yersin became himself, finally managing to shuck off the carapace of shyness and social awkwardness that weighed so heavy on him in Europe. Among people who knew nothing of science nor Paris, nor the pressures exerted on the young white man by ambitious family, Yersin flowered. He became charming, candid, humorous, relaxed. Gone was the weary boy of Paris, who'd confided morosely in his mother that he only liked one painting in the Louvre, and that for its 'desolation and sadness'; in his place was an explorer in the Livingstone cast, effortlessly courageous, able to see beyond the jingoistic posturings of his colonial overlords to the humanity in each situation and confrontation.

To begin with, his forays into the interior of Vietnam – funded by a French government anxious to map the unknown interiors of its colonial possessions – were restricted to his periods of ship doctor's shore leave. This was a job he held for only a year before, in December 1891, being made a colonial doctor, a post which offered almost endless scope for exploration. And it was for these escapes – becoming the first European to penetrate the mountains; struggling to find porters bold enough to risk facing both pirates and the leeches; the adrenaline rush of knowing that, any night, they might be the object of rebel attack – that, increasingly, he lived. By contrast, the quotidian grind of doctoring began to irritate. To his mother he wrote: 'You ask me if I have developed a taste for medical practice. Yes and no. I have great pleasure in curing people who come to see me but I don't really want to become a doctor, to make money out of being a doctor . . . I find it vile and repugnant to ask money for curing people. It's a bit like saying, "Your money or your life".'

The maps he made during these Vietnam journeys of the early 1890s were painstaking and topographically impressive, and were seized upon by contemporary geographers. On each return from the wilderness he was pushed for intelligence, the latest news on tribal rivalries, for descriptions of mountain ranges and river courses that no other white man had ever seen. Faced with such respect – as in June 1892, when he dined with the French governor in Phnom Penh – Yersin appeared genuinely nonplussed, rather than calculatedly over-modest. 'Everyone here,' he told his mother, even as he digested the governor's foie gras, 'thinks I've done an extraordinary trip. I really don't believe it was that special. No one seems to believe that I've lived two months on rice alone and yet the indigenous population are forced to live on rice.'

These were years of tempering, a distillation of his essence, a necessary preparation for all that was to come. In June 1893, deep in the interior, he surprised a cache of anti-colonial rebels, an ambush that resulted in Yersin singlehandedly fending off the outlaws while his men fled into the jungle. Recovering in hospital, his spirit unbroken, Yersin began to plan his next foray. This was his biggest-ever expedition, at the head of a team of seventy porters and soldiers, a journey which would last some three months, and during which, on account of an unexplained village fire, he would be accused of witchcraft and once again only just manage to escape with his life.

He remains a conundrum, an amalgam of the heroic and the clumsy, a man who could face up to bandits but who found even the smallest cocktail party an insufferable ordeal, for whom one rejection in love was enough to warn him off women for life. He was complex, often unfathomable even to his friends. Yet the eight-year-old capable of a chilling degree of forensic detachment would become a man of honour and courage, absolutely loyal. He was a fierce patriot and was born at a time when colonial excesses were at their most pernicious, yet was never heard to denigrate another on grounds of race or skin colour. During one period of doctoring he was robbed continually by his patients, yet found it impossible to condemn. 'We the French have always stolen from the people in Indochina, so it might be quite good that they can steal a bit of my money back.'

All this, and only thirty years old: for most people, even the most adventurous of his contemporaries, such achievements would have been enough for eighty years.

*

THEN, IN THE FIRST months of 1894, bubonic plague hit Hong Kong, the world's fourth largest merchant and passenger port, a British colony. Plague, which had destroyed the European population during the fourteenth century – and had exploded in sporadic, ferocious outbreaks ever since – had returned, and at the very moment when medicine was beginning to grow complacent, to congratulate itself on the progress achieved so far in the war against disease.

Worse still, there was no cure. Terrified plague would escape from Hong Kong and that in time nowhere would be safe, the island government appealed for help. For the Pasteur Institute in Paris, only one researcher would do. Yersin may have been young, but few possessed the kind of bravery and clearsightedness he had already demonstrated. On 12 June 1894 he set sail from Saigon, Hong Kong-bound.

Chapter One

No DISEASE in recorded history has carried the totemic power of plague. No disease has erupted with such violence and eradicated populations so quickly and with such brutal efficiency, nor remained so poorly understood for so long. Plague is the archetypal horror-flick killer, with the bore-hole-black eyes of the serial murderer, the passionless brutality, the questing and insatiable thirst for destruction. Plague has inspired more literature than any other epidemic, has set humans against each other in a way only normally witnessed during the darkest hours of war. It has transcended itself to become emblematic of something far more invasive and apocalyptic than mere infection; the word itself – *plague* – deserves a paragraph all its own, to be printed in twenty-six-point type, a warning in and of itself. Time has made it more: a collective noun for any malevolent force – locusts, warplanes, hurricane rains – and a verb for the worst that one person can do to another, to plague being to torment, to drive insane.

For centuries, the disease was so feared that 'plague' as an uttered word, as a single quiet syllable, was held to carry a unique power. Simply to murmur it risked unleashing the infection and so, in 1745, Frederick the Great forbade his generals from using the word, insisting instead on the gentler, less panic-inducing 'foul fever'. Leading the French invasion of Egypt in 1798, Napoleon Bonaparte went further: not only were mentions of plague outlawed, but, when the illness tore through his troops at Alexandria, he could be seen bending over sickbeds in the lazaretto in Jaffa, touching the hands of the afflicted, like Princess Diana embracing men gaunt and liverish with Aids: look at me, he was saying, look how little I am alarmed, how benign this disease you so fear. Later, pseudonyms grew ever more various, more unlikely: 'typhoid pneumonia', 'croupous pneumonia', 'intermittent fever'.

Most commonly, plague has been explained as an act of God, a punishment for wickedness and shortcoming. To the credulous and superstitious Europeans of the Middle Ages, the ravages of the mid-fourteenth century pandemic, the Black Death, were just retribution for any number of transgressions: heresy, lechery, avarice, episcopal decadence, the greed of kings, the drunkenness of the peasantry. And for those whose neighbourhoods remained plague-free almost anything was quakingly read as portent: heavy mist, falling stars, blasts of hot wind from the south, blood spots on freshly baked bread, a stranded whale.

Ignorance about the causes of plague created a vacuum through which wildly competing theories coursed, each with their vigorous and persuasive proponents, their noisy gain-sayers. In the Middle Ages, thought was split: plague could be caught either from another person or from a 'miasma', a kind of atmospheric corruption. This was an infinitely broad and accommodating category, and consequently the most popular: corruption of the air was believed to be caused either by organic decay or by such natural calamities as earthquakes or noxious gases escaping from fissures in the ground. For those who held that contagion spread person to person, the only security lay in isolation. Safest of all, if a certain physician from Montpellier was to be believed, was to remain blindfolded throughout the epidemic: 'Instantaneous death occurs when the aerial spirit escaping from the eyes of the sick man strikes the eyes of a healthy person standing near and looking at the sick, especially when the latter are in agony.'

Each time plague reared up again, this centuries-old controversy was revived. By the nineteenth century the two camps were no closer to agreement, and an outbreak from 1834 to 1835 – which claimed 32,000 lives as it spread from Alexandria to Cairo – triggered a spate of medical publications from Europe's most respected physicians. Records survive of one doctor – a stalwart of the contagionist school – who never ventured out during the epidemic without a posse of four mounted servants to protect him from chance contact with plague cases. He wore a protective suit with a mantle of oilcloth, and covered his saddle with waxed material. When diagnosing and treating patients, he made sure never to touch their bare skin, preferring instead to dip his fingers in oil, wrap them in tobacco leaves, and only then to attempt to feel the pulse. His best efforts notwithstanding, he was dead of plague within the year.

Most physicians' attempts to understand plague amounted to little more than wild fumblings, their theories born more of prejudice and fear than educated calculation. For millennia – through the pandemics of the sixth and fourteenth centuries, through countless more localized epidemics – the disease had maintained absolute supremacy, a fixed point around which scientists and doctors flailed blindly, inventing ever more preposterous experiments to prove their hypotheses.

In the 1830s, during the Egyptian outbreak, French advocates of the contagionist theory devised a series of trials that, had they been conducted today, would have caused severing of diplomatic relations, trade embargoes, petitions to United Nations human rights committees. In one experiment, a condemned criminal was injected with pus from a plague bubo and his progress thereafter closely monitored. His continued good health must have cheered the next criminal to be plucked from death row, since all this unfortunate had to do was sleep in a hospital cot in which another had died of plague. When, shortly afterwards, he developed the listless fever, the blood-stained sputum, the bloated and cyanosed face common to all plague victims, the scientists claimed proof: here was a disease propagated by putrefaction; the only quicker way to contract it would have been to lie alongside the decaying corpse itself.

By the late nineteenth century, the field had become crowded: with no empirical research in place, and no proven technique or concrete lead, the proponents of all competing theories held equal sway. Having made little headway since the fourteenth century, authorities – depending on religious or cultural persuasion – explained plague as an infection brought on by any one of the following: the wrath of God, corruption of the air or soil, overcrowding and filth, a general or specific moral laxity, a straightforward person-to-person contagion, a particular alignment of stars, a stifling climate, or proximity to putrefying corpses, as in the case of the vaults and catacombs of Cairo, where the annual Nile floods saw body parts washed past bathers, washerwomen and children splashing in the shallows.

Methods of prevention were as various as the causes: judiciously worn dried toads, amulets filled with arsenic, lockets containing camphor or eucalyptus. However, the safest and simplest of all the means of warding off plague, according to brothers George and John Thomson – working in Bombay in the early 1900s, as the Hong Kong plague turned global – was to throw open the window. The 'virulence of the germ', they claimed, was neutralized by a 'sufficiency of fresh air'.

Scientific memory can be woefully short. By the 1890s, plague had been almost forgotten, part of the folklore of Dark Age horrors. Since 1835, with the end of the Egyptian outbreak, there had been only sporadic and limited episodes, meagre enough in scale and effect to relegate plague to the lower division of dangerous diseases. So the news from southern China and Hong Kong in the late spring of 1894 that plague was resurgent came not only as a powerful jolt – a sickening sense, as with approaching war, that boundaries and all the best human efforts counted for nothing – but as the ultimate challenge: of all diseases, plague was the most dreaded. The wake-up call from Hong Kong proved the spur to a heroic and largely forgotten scientific endeavour and one that, moreover, resonates powerfully today. Even now plague is a disease that, as in the quiet years before 1894, is – in the words of one contemporary frontline researcher – merely dormant, 'down but not out'.

Chapter Two

IN THE FIFTEENTH *arrondissement* of Paris, deep in the basement archives of the Pasteur Institute in rue du Docteur
Roux, lies a manuscript which, in twenty-five densely hand-
written pages, tells an extraordinary, heroic story. *Mon Voyage
à Hong Kong au Sujet de la Peste* is Yersin's unpublished memoir
of his fight – against the might of the colonial authorities,
against competing scientists – to track down the cause of
plague. Around him in Hong Kong, as the summer heat
of 1894 thickened, the disease raged unchecked; by 1910, it
would have spread to India, Bolivia, Australia and the west
coast of America, claiming many millions of lives. Yersin's
goal – the cure for a disease that had caused more devastation than any other in history – was the most ambitious
imaginable.

*

YERSIN'S PACKET BOAT docked in Hong Kong harbour
on 15 June 1894. In the five weeks since plague had been
confirmed and the deaths had begun escalating, the colony
had been transformed. Where before had been the constant
motion of liveried porters unloading trunks from visitors as
far afield as America, Singapore, London and Japan, now
there was unholy quiet, customs posts manned by skeleton
crews, the only quayside movement visible from the deck

of an approaching ship the slow shuffle-onward of coffin-bearers, heads down, shoulders bowed, feet dragging eddies of dust.

From ebullience to fear, confidence to suspicion, neighbour against neighbour, European against Chinese. Hong Kong in 1894, though only fifty-three years into its colonial role, was already a port of international significance and renown: from two thousand fishermen in 1841, this 'barren rock' so comprehensively damned by Britain's Foreign Secretary Lord Palmerston had become home to a hundred times that. Writers of tourist guidebooks spoke wonderingly of the 'pleasant but mild excitement combined with feelings of contentment and security' that the fortunate visitor would experience when first approaching the island. Hoteliers, fully aware of the colony's attractions, clambered over one another to pull in custom. The Hong Kong Hotel, overlooking Victoria harbour, boasted 'Hydraulic Ascending Rooms of the latest and most approved type'; for the Windsor Hotel, the draw was the architecture – 'finest in the colony' – and the cuisine – 'under European supervision'.

Most Europeans, however, paid scant attention to either the landscape or the hotels' décor: for them, a Hong Kong posting was part of a carefully judged career strategy. For Sir William Goodman, who would become Chief Justice of the Hong Kong Supreme Court, the decision to leave a respectable but unremarkable bar practice in the London suburbs and 'look for some appointment in the Colonies' was down to an 'anxiousness about my professional outlook'. For the young James Stewart Lockhart, setting sail for Hong Kong in 1879, the expectation was of fortunes to be made, claims staked, just as several of his Argyll relatives had done in the colony before him. Like Goodman, Lockhart was methodical in his ambition: two years in Guangzhou to study Cantonese – the necessary leg-up over monolingual colleagues – before his first Hong Kong government appointment. By 1894, the year plague struck, he would be Acting Colonial Secretary, struggling to keep order when all around was panic, flight, mob violence.

The life led by the colonial overlords was leisured and gracious, if socially restricted. The European upper classes mixed neither with other whites of lesser social standing, nor with the Chinese. Instead – for reasons of climate as much as snobbery – they retreated uphill, to the cool mountainous slopes overlooking the harbour, where they built great veranda'd mansions and shady arboretums. Here, in the 'Peak District', on vast sprinklered lawns, in front of stuccoed palaces, lifting tumblers of freshly squeezed lemonade from silver trays, women in white dresses spent the afternoons playing croquet. Their children – those not yet old enough to have been dispatched by steamer to boarding school in England – trailed in silent crocodiles along paths sheltered from the midday sun by camphor and high citrus trees, governesses at front and back. Come evening, with the children asleep, there would be dinner parties, concerts, bridge fours: the same faces uttering similar platitudes, with only the electric rattle of insects just beyond the screen doors to break the spell, to remind them that they were not in fact home in comfortable Dorking or Harrow.

The maintenance of European life and custom was an uncertain process, and involved a good degree of wishful thinking. For as long as they kept themselves loftily separate on the slopes of the Peak, the Europeans could persuade themselves the other world did not exist: the Hong Kong of crowded tenement housing, where animals slept in the same rooms as their masters, where cholera was a constant menace, where a combination of careless and insanitary living, serious overcrowding, and a high rat population was fast creating the perfect breeding ground for plague.

Of the white population, only the working man had intercourse with the Chinese: it was the footsoldier or wharf labourer who frequented Chinese brothels; the bureaucrats and office workers, businessmen and more senior military ranks invested their surplus pay with European or American prostitutes.

When they grew tired of whoring, on-leave sailors and merchant seamen caroused their way through central Hong Kong, staggering from door to door, throwing money at whichever householder had alcohol to sell. Like wayward magnets, they were attracted most often to the island's least salubrious quarter, the all-Chinese Taipingshan, an area so famously insanitary that, when plague erupted there in the spring of 1894, it was impossible for anyone to feign surprise. Through here, throughout the small hours, dishevelled ships' crews of all nationalities danced chaotically to the hornpipe, hollering out some rough approximation of a sea shanty. Their arrival in port was dreaded by resident Europeans, and no doubt by most Chinese. 'They drink like fishes,' lamented a Wesleyan missionary just weeks before plague broke out. 'They ride around in rickshaws, making the night hideous with their shouts, eat overripe fruit from street stalls, are stricken with cholera, and die in a few hours.'

In their drive for self-obliteration, these incautious revellers failed to notice the fatigue and resignation on the faces of the Chinese serving them, who silently offered shot glasses of hooch and, just as quietly, palmed the proffered dollars. For behind the doorways in which they stood were buildings in which no European – of however humble birth or expectation – would ever have countenanced living.

Taipingshan covered ten acres: 384 scrappily built brick houses wedged against a sharply sloping hillside, the 'Great Peace Mountain'. Because of the incline, the back of the ground floor of each dwelling was subterranean, and therefore windowless; the floor was of earth, and often damp. Above were two, sometimes three storeys, the floors of which were fitted with rough boards through which detritus, liquid and dust fell freely, and it was in box partitions in these upper rooms that nine or ten whole families would bed down: five or six individuals at a time, children and a cross-section of generations and all their possessions, shoehorned into a space twelve feet square. Rooms over fourteen feet high were subdivided both vertically and horizontally, a practice which not only provided another floor but also cast into sepulchral darkness the partitions and families below. With no chimney, the air was opaque and choking with cooking smoke, the atmosphere hot and foetid from the smouldering urns of pig fat, rendered from hogs which, deprived of their own rooting space, spent their short lives making their sties in the bedrooms of their owners. What water there was came from wells that even the Chinese considered hazardous to health. In short: an entire district that was not only a potent reservoir of everyday illness, but a place where contagion, once started, would prove impossible to stop.

Yet, over the years, there had been warning voices. As early as 1851, only a decade into the colony's life, the colonial surgeon was using his annual report to lament

the 'dirty and gregarious habits of the people and the pestilential defects in the construction and situation of their
dwellings'. Twenty-one years later, the new appointee to the
post, Dr Philip Ayres, found that little had changed: brothels
were breeding typhoid; Chinese houses, the construction of
which flouted 'every rule', were 'not fit for pigs'; most
sewage drains were simply allowed to peter out at the end
of the street, excreta leeching into the subsoil. Yet, again,
no action was taken: Ayres himself, due to opium addiction,
was held to be an unreliable witness and his report was
buried.

By 1882, when Osbert Chadwick from London's Institute of Civil Engineers was sent to Hong Kong expressly
to study and report back on the worsening overcrowding
and attendant, chaotic sanitation, conditions had deterio-
rated to a point where language almost failed him. 'The
system of house drainage,' he sighed, 'is radically bad.'
There was a bare handful of public latrines, the water
supply was inadequate, what sewage that made it to
drainage culverts ended up straight in the harbour. Government should shake itself to action, he counselled. 'My report
will show the necessity for strong and complete measures
of sanitation, and I trust that they will be undertaken for
the immediate benefit of the public health without waiting
for the necessity to be demonstrated by the irresistible logic
of an epidemic.'

Despite the mounting evidence in favour of a radical
clean-up, the next few years were marked by bureaucratic
procrastination, not decisive action: the passing of a public
health ordinance; the appointment of a sanitation board,
then endless arguments over its scope and power; then yet
more ordinances and the insertion of careful subsidiary

clauses, followed by yet another sanitation study. The 'unreliable' Dr Ayres, after an 1893 house inspection, sounded close to despair: 'The floors were reeking with filth. The drainage was very bad, the smell abominable. In some of the houses were dark holes in which there were quantities of decomposing and putrid meat, fat and bones, and one of them filled with maggots. The stench was unbearable. I found [these houses] in the same condition I had reported twenty years ago.'

The cumulative effect of decades of unheeded warnings was a kind of collective numbness among the European population, an indifference heightened by the fact that, during the same period, their own health and sanitation had steadily improved. The numbers being invalided home were falling, streets in the white districts were wider and drainage more efficient. With this came confidence, long afternoons whiled away at the Happy Valley racecourse, evenings at the Hong Kong Jockey Club. For government officials and doctors, civil engineers and town planners, for all those who had so effectively silenced their professional consciences, the life of these last days was an easeful, leisured existence.

Few partied harder than the most senior doctor of all, James Lowson, Superintendent of the showpiece Government Civil Hospital, a giant white-porticoed monolith on the lower slopes of the Peak. Entries in his diary are brief, often costive, but preciously illuminative of this life of the privileged classes. The year started busy, as it would continue. On Saturday 6 January 1894, Lowson, one of the colony's most gifted sportsmen, wrote, 'Cricket. Made 107 + 3 for 23. Maxim Gun Corps.' A week later he was skippering 'Stella, Paddy May's yacht ... came in first'.

There were golf tournaments, balls, nightly dinner parties, all of them noted. Friends and acquaintances were mentioned in often cursory fashion, with some abruptness, surnames only: 'Atkinson left at 5.30 for Canton with Pearson and his womenkind.' The flippancy discernible in that 'womenkind' is evident elsewhere: in his description of an acquaintance being accidentally knocked over by a gun as 'amusing'; in his free admission to another that he 'did not care a tinker's dam [sic] for him'; in his dismissal of the suffering of yet another with the perfunctory 'tired of life – cheer up'.

Lowson was at the top of the colonial ladder and so, when plague was first reported over the border at Canton, he would have known that this, of all medical matters, was not something happily left to a subordinate: he'd have had no choice but to investigate personally. On Saturday 5 May, a day when he would normally have been contentedly pulling on his cricket whites in preparation for a weekend at the crease, he was in Canton, conferring with worried local doctors. By Monday, he was back in Hong Kong, where rumour had preceded him, and there was little he could do to stifle speculation. Plague had leapt the Chinese border. The Black Death was back. The world was no longer safe.

Chapter Three

JAMES ALFRED LOWSON was still two months short of his twenty-eighth birthday when he made his first, reluctant diagnosis of plague. From photographs he appears older, tougher-skinned, suspicious. In one, the closest to an unposed snapshot that survives, he sits on the edge of what looks like a hotel bed, possibly in Canton during that first long plague weekend.

The shot has a spontaneous, rickety feel. He is wearing a silk jacket, in style a Western–Chinese hybrid, with Chinese bobble fasteners in place of buttons, and a V-cut, Savile Row collar. His legs are crossed, hands folded in his lap. His hair is combed flat to his head, with a rigid, straight-ruled parting. He wears a long, downangled moustache and is looking over the photographer's shoulder, at a point high up, near the ceiling. In certain immediate ways he is unusual-looking, and it is not hard to imagine how those misaligned eyes, that sour-fruit mouth, could make an outsider feel profoundly ill-at-ease and unwelcome, the fumbling gatecrasher.

On Monday 7 May 1894, Lowson and his fellow investigators climbed aboard the ferry that would return them from Canton, down the Pearl River, to Hong Kong. They arrived back that afternoon. 'In club at 6 p.m.,' his diary reads. 'Rumours of plague.' In the early hours of Tuesday, rumour became fact, with Lowson's positive Hong Kong identification. '1 a.m. diagnosed A. Hung as suffering from the plague and isolated him.'

*

EXACTLY ONE WEEK LATER, Yersin – ignorant of the escalating emergency in Hong Kong – arrived in Saigon, anticipating a long and much needed period of rest. The previous three months had seen the most ambitious and gruelling of his expeditions so far, an exploration of the uncharted region between Nha-Trang and Tourane. During those weeks he had passed through lands belonging to tribes who had never before seen a white man, many of whose people had, fearing diabolical, pale-skinned witchcraft, barricaded their village gates against his approach. The report he handed to the colonial authorities was notable for its balance and restraint – despite its author's ordeal – and was also rich in detail, analysis, description: of the topography of the plains and mountains, of the customs and beliefs of each tribe he encountered, of the possibility of a colossal haul of gold, of the need for a fairer system of tax.

From the report, one gets the impression of a young man bent on extreme exploration, as obsessed by geographical exactitude as by notions of racial fairness. With his letters home, though, the focus narrows: his 'dream', he tells his mother, is to 'follow the trail of Livingstone'. Yet, during this time, Yersin was, through official channels, pursuing a quite separate goal.

For at least forty years, plague had been a constant menace in the southern states of China – flaring up, then abating, never quite disappearing. As early as 1850, the *Overland Friend of China*, an old-school colonial newspaper, reported that Canton 'and the neighbouring towns and villages are afflicted by a malignant fever . . . [that] resembles the plague which desolated London two centuries ago . . . We are in hopes that it will not extend to Europeans.' More detail, of a more measured kind, was forthcoming in 1889, with the publication of the British Government's *Imperial Maritime Customs' Annual Report*, which claimed that Yunnan province, northwest of Canton, had 'suffered annually for a period of years from the plague, a kind of malignant fever, fatal in a few days, having as one of its symptoms a hard swelling on the neck, in the armpits, or in the groin'. Rats and cattle were conspicuous casualties; immunity, apparently, was conferred by altitude: plague 'rarely scales heights over 7,200 feet high'.

Ever since his arrival in Indochina in 1892, Yersin – in common with every alert traveller – had been aware of the presence of plague in the region. Within weeks of his arrival, he was petitioning the French Governor-General, Jean-Marie de Lanessan, requesting permission to leave for Yunnan to study the disease: clearly, he told de Lanessan, himself a former doctor, prompt action was required. He could start, he pledged, as soon as he returned from his first, eagerly anticipated, journey into the Vietnamese interior.

The response from de Lanessan was swift and brutal, a breathtaking demonstration of how far behind he'd left his Hippocratic roots. 'There has never been plague in Yunnan,' he replied flatly. 'And if there were, I would deny it. We put poor old Tonkin [the northernmost region of Vietnam, bordering China's Yunnan province] down enough without laying plague at its door as well.'

Yersin, running short of time before the start of his expedition, and powerless against such determined and

high-level resistance, quietly withdrew, aware that another
angle of attack was needed. In fact, as he later wrote in his
notes for the Pasteur Institute, 'Plague was no longer raging
exclusively in Yunnan, but had reached Long-Tcheou and
Pakhoï . . . the whole frontier of Tonkin was threatened.'
However, alone, he could not supply sufficient leverage:
to de Lanessan, intent above all on short-term political
expediency, on the diplomacy of minimum offence, Yersin
– with his irritating whine about some obscure, long-dead
disease – was as a persistent mosquito, a trivial distraction
from the real business of government.

Away in the mountains, at the start of a four-month
trek that would take him some two hundred miles from
coastal Nha-Trang, inland through jungle ranges to the
Mekong, then down the great sweeping caramel river to
Phnom Penh, Yersin's determination was hardening.
Laboratory life, he now knew, was not for him: 'My firm
intention is never again to work at the Pasteur Institute.
I spent enough time there . . . and now that I am far
away, I can judge it more objectively. Life in a laboratory
would seem impossible to me after having tasted the
freedom and life of the open air.'

Moreover, it is clear from the laconic tone of his letters
that physical danger never once threatened to overwhelm
him – as it might have done with a more normal, more
fearful man. Days when his party was attacked are detailed
precisely, but without notable emotion. Events unfold, speak
for themselves, are almost comic in their understatement.
On 24 June 1893, high up in the mountains, he and his
men set off after a band of rebels 'armed with machetes,
spears and rifles' whose plan, Yersin learned, was to massacre the French in Phan Rang. 'Of course,' he writes, 'I

had to act.' A day later, his own men once again having
fled, Yersin not for the first time found himself alone with
the enemy. Runs his deadpan summation: 'I only [now] had
to fight the five chiefs.' His success resulted in the rebel
leader's execution, which Yersin was invited to watch.
'Beyond any doubt,' he would write, the execution of Thouk
'was a gruesome sight. His head fell after the fourth sabre
blow. [He] did not even budge. These Annamese die with
a truly impressive coolness.'

*

BY OCTOBER 1893, Yersin was back in Saigon and gearing
up for another assault on the Governor-General. This
time, however, he was armed with fresh intelligence: word
had reached him that, during his absence, de Lanessan had
received an unequivocal ministerial dispatch from Paris,
ordering him to send a plague researcher to Yunnan. All
Yersin had to do was put himself forward.

Buoyed by this information, Yersin would have arrived
in confident mood for his audience with the Governor-
General. Since his return from the mountains he'd become
something of a celebrity in the colonial capital, his heroic,
singlehanded defeat of Thouk's rebels discussed in awed
tones at dinner parties, in the marketplace, on the croquet
lawn. In turn, Yersin was growing visibly in presence and
confidence: the shy young man of Paris, diffident in the
company of his peers, had been transformed. For the first
time in his life – many thousands of miles and a whole new
culture from the land of his birth – he felt at home.

Yet, despite the orders from Paris, his meeting with the
Governor-General resulted in as much frustration as before.

De Lanessan, who had first questioned even the existence of plague, now used cost as his reason for obstruction.

'Who,' he demanded, 'will pay the bill?'

'The colony,' replied Yersin, who had no reason to believe any different, and whose astonishment at the Governor-General's reaction was such that he recorded the exchange verbatim in his official report. 'The colony would cover it, I would think.'

'You think that,' de Lanessan shot back, 'then you are wrong. You are very wrong.'

*

FEW NEWS STORIES, from any age, have excited journalists more than an outbreak of plague, and it took less than twenty-four hours for the first Hong Kong reporter to catch wind of James Lowson's initial reluctant diagnosis. By midday on 9 May 1894, there would have been no one in the colony ignorant of the *Telegraph*'s front-page bulletin. 'A fatal disease,' the paper announced, 'somewhat similar in its effects to the "black fever", which has carried off thousands of the natives of Canton during the past month . . . has, we regret to learn, made its appearance among the Chinese residents in the Taipingshan district.'

Few diseases have ever been more feared and so it was only inevitable that those with the most to lose should be the quickest to voice denials. According to the *Telegraph*, the government, in the person of the Registrar of Deaths, had moved swiftly to quash any mention of plague, 'courteously informing us that the deaths in Taipingshan district today are . . . from diarrhoea, phthisis, bronchitis, etc.; none from plague.' Such, however, was the reliability of the paper's source that this was not the last word. 'In Chinese circles,' the report concluded, 'the existence of a very fatal disease of some kind in Taipingshan is insisted upon.'

A day later, with panic rising in the crowded Chinese quarter, the government was resolutely sticking to its story. On 10 May, the *Hong Kong Daily Press*, without any discernible hint of irony, reported some forty deaths in Taipingshan in the previous two days, a mortality rate that the authorities apparently judged unremarkable. 'On enquiry with the Registrar-General's department, we find that no suspicious deaths have been reported, and that no information has been received – although enquiries were carried out – which justifies any apprehension that an epidemic is likely to break out.'

For much of the mid-nineteenth century – from 1851, a decade after the birth of the colony, till the early 1870s – the Hong Kong Chinese, in their treatment of terminal illness, had unwittingly done pretty much all they could to breed sickness. The worst such example was the I-ts'z, a temple-cum-death house in the centre of Taipingshan: behind the shroud of blue incense in the main hall were eight cubicles, rented out to the families of the dying, where, in garments gone cheesy with sweat and faeces, unattended by any kind of regular doctor, the sick would wait for death.

To the Chinese, few things were guaranteed to confer uncleanliness more effectively than proximity to someone close to death: hence the I-ts'z, where the dying were abandoned. It took the colonial authorities a good eighteen years to register properly the inhumanity and full medical horror of the I-ts'z and that only by chance, during the course of an investigation into the death of a valued worker from the emigration depot who had expired in the sub-Dickensian squalor in the spring of 1869.

The dubious honour of recording the gruesomeness of
the I-ts'z fell to Alfred Lister, Registrar General. 'At my first
visit there were, dead and alive, about nine or ten patients
in the so-called hospital. One, apparently dying from emaci-
ation and diarrhoea, was barricaded into a place just large
enough to hold the board on which he lay, and not high
enough to stand up in, another room contained a boarding
on which lay two poor creatures half-dead, and one corpse,
while the floor, which was of earth, was covered in pools
of urine. The next room contained what the attendants
asserted to be two corpses, but on examination one of
them was found to be alive . . . the other rooms contained
miserable and emaciated creations, unable to speak or
move, whose rags had apparently never been changed since
their admission, and whom the necessities of nature had
reduced to an inexpressibly sickening condition.'

Lister's revelations had repercussions far beyond the
slew of ghoulish headlines in the next morning's papers.
Within the ranks of the colonial bureaucracy, the search
for a scapegoat was immediately triggered; when the news
reached London, it was held up as further evidence of the
abuses of the 'coolie trade'. Policemen stormed the I-ts'z,
removed the dead and sent those still breathing to the
Government Civil Hospital. They then forbade the building
to be used as anything other than a temple, a ruling which
led to a build-up of corpses and the dying on street corners,
of bodies abandoned and putrescent, aswarm with crawling
things, slimy with decay.

The governor at the time, Richard MacDonnell,
ordered action: specifically, a hospital set up for and funded
by the Chinese. Fundraising would not be a problem, he
believed; for evidence of the 'great wealth' of the Hong

Kong Chinese, one need look no further than the large
sums spent on 'their puerile national processions and
"shows" every year'. The Chinese, for their part, chose to
overlook the governor's slight and stumped up $47,000 –
three times the amount MacDonnell had hoped for – to
which the government added a further $115,000.

*

THE TUNG WAH HOSPITAL – treating patients with traditional Chinese methods, eschewing the Western model in
every detail right down to its accounting methods – opened
in February 1872. For the first time in Hong Kong, Chinese
medicine was made respectable, even establishment. At the
Tung Wah, as on most street corners, treatment was with
herbs, the philosophy one of balance: between Yin and
Yang, a disequilibrium of which would spark disease. The
organs were classified according to the five elements of the
universe – gold for the lung, wood for the liver, water for
the kidney, fire for the heart and earth for the stomach and
spleen – and could react with each other in the same way
as the elements themselves. It was a system distinguished
above all by curiosities: feeling the pulse, the most important of all diagnostic practices, was impossible with a non-
consenting female patient and so a length of string would
be tied around her wrist; the doctor, holding the other end,
would somehow manage to gauge her well-being. For the
Western physician witnessing such eccentricities, the reaction was invariably the same: to Dr Philip Ayres Chinese
methods were 'nothing but empiricism and quackery'.

Much the same could have been fairly said of the kind
of practices adopted by Dr Ayres and colleagues. When
plague hit, the European doctors – all the while brazenly

boasting of their expertise and their pre-eminence in the face of rampant infection – adopted a sweeping approach that spoke most eloquently about the extent of their ignorance. Furniture was burned, clothing soaked in Jeyes Fluid disinfectant, interior walls whitewashed; eventually, nothing but wholesale demolition of the plague district was deemed sufficient. Hardly surprising, in short, that the Tung Wah Hospital should have been driven to the point where it found itself encouraging open rebellion against the government, a move which led to swift retaliation: the mooring of a fully armed gunboat just offshore, its cannons trained on the roof of the Chinese hospital.

Chapter Four

A SOLDIER WITH a box camera stands at the top of a narrow back alley. Below him, halfway down the sharp incline, between houses shuttered and barred, are ten others: sleeves rolled up, white helmets brilliant in the heat, smoking pipes to disguise the stench of the work. The soldier raises the camera to his eye, composes the shot. As he presses the shutter, he thinks: this could be home, that old Chinese woman looking on dismayed as her clothes are plunged in disinfectant my own grandmother, the street itself a slum in any northern town. Yet it feels reassuringly foreign, too, and the plague he and his fellow military are engaged in fighting so clearly the product of oriental neglect and slatternly Chinese housekeeping. They deserve all this, he figures, as he slips his camera into his pocket and reaches for his broom, roused to action by the sudden hollering of the colour sergeant – all this intrusion, their homes turned upside-down, the forced entry and eviction. They should consider themselves lucky.

What the soldier and the three hundred or so other plague fighters from the Shropshire Light Infantry did not know was that already, less than a week into the epidemic, something close to panic was infecting high command. Safe in the cocoon of his orders – to search every house, douse clothing and bedding and furniture with disinfectant, to ignore any plea or protestation from the householders – the soldier would have been unaware of the wild fumbling that distinguished the government's first attempts at curbing the spread of disease. On 11 May, two days after the first apocalyptic headline, James Lowson and Philip Ayres – the colony's most senior doctors, and a pair united in their distaste for political double-speak – were called as witnesses before an extraordinary meeting of the sanitary board. Their joint report detailed their visit the day before to the Tung Wah hospital, where they'd rooted out no less than twenty cases of plague. Yet still – despite Lowson's first-hand witness from Canton, where he'd seen the hospitals filled to their entrance halls with the moaning and feverish, all displaying identical symptoms to those now dying in Hong Kong – the committee chairman remained sceptically aloof. Throughout, he studiously avoided using of the word 'plague', as if just to utter it might bring it into being. Instead, the transcripts show him opting for laborious euphemisms: 'epidemic', 'endemic disease', 'contagious disease'.

He need not have bothered. Fearing Chinese reprisals at the forced 'cleansing' of their homes, European doctors had taken to carrying revolvers on their rounds, their pockets weighty and percussive with shells. In New York, Buenos Aires and London, owners of shipping lines were tracing nervous fingers across the maritime charts, looking at alternative Far Eastern harbours: Shanghai, Saigon, Manila. The word was out: Hong Kong was unsafe, had become within the space of days a leprous brother, excluded from the international family.

It must have been at least in part an effort at wresting back some measure of control that led Sir William Robinson, governor of the colony for the last three years, to put out a plea for help. Plague was looming unmanageable, that much he could see, and despite their bold assertions to the contrary, his own doctors clearly understood little of its mechanics, causes, or how it spread. To his cry for assistance the world's finest responded: Professor Shibasaburo Kitasato, celebrated already for his discovery of the tetanus bacillus; and Dr Alexandre Yersin, explorer of the dark Indochinese interior, diphtheria pioneer, and as rough-edged a maverick as Kitasato was sleek, proper and establishment.

The two men were similar in only one regard: the quality of their professional commitment and dedication. Kitasato was older and, from photographs taken during his time in Hong Kong, appears a somewhat dour forty-two-year-old; the thirty-one-year-old Yersin, by contrast, seems serious, but not without some humility, some sense of his place in things. One snapshot shows the Japanese and eight European doctors, posed as if for a team photograph, Kitasato sitting right in the centre. More than anything, the photograph speaks of the welcome Kitasato – or 'The Professor', as the colony's newspaper would deferentially refer to him – received from Hong Kong's foremost physicians. Flanking the lone Japanese are Ayres, the extravagantly moustachioed colonial surgeon, Lowson, Kitasato's greatest champion and ally, and six other top surgeons and doctors. What pervades is an air of quiet self-congratulation, embodied in Kitasato's slouched pose, the way his head is tilted back and his eyes seem half closed, the straw boater at rest casually in his lap, fingertips caressing the brim.

To European eyes, accustomed to the slighter build of most Chinese, Kitasato was comically stocky, even freakish.

One newspaper, early on, before his celebrity was fully established, pictured him as 'a short-haired and profound-looking gentleman with a very large head'. On the few occasions that he made the news, Yersin was either 'the Frenchman', 'Dr Yersin' or, with icy sarcasm, the '*savant*'. Despite his outsized cranium, it was Kitasato whose personality, appearance and professional approach most appealed to the Hong Kong establishment. Not being French – and thus removed from the region's intense Anglo-French colonial rivalry – was of course an advantage, as no doubt was his penchant for the severely formal uniform of starched white collar and morning coat in the laboratory. To Lowson, who hosted him regularly at dinner, Kitasato was a 'good chap'. Praise seldom came much higher than this.

He was also a formidable scientific intellect. Born in 1852 in a mountain village in southern Japan, he would become one of his country's first and most celebrated microbiologists. In 1886, at the age of thirty-three, Kitasato, then working for the Japanese government, was picked as the first foreigner to travel to Berlin to study under the genius tutelage of Robert Koch. The extension of his stay from three to six years was due to Koch's personal intervention: so groundbreaking had been Kitasato's work on tuberculosis that Koch successfully petitioned the Emperor of Japan for Kitasato to be allowed to stay on. His return to Japan in 1892 was equally auspicious: before leaving Koch's laboratory, the German government awarded him the title of professor, the first such honour ever accorded a foreign scientist.

Kitasato set sail from Japan less than a week after his government received Hong Kong's mayday. A substantial expedition was assembled, gathering excitedly on the Tokyo quayside, surrounded by trunks of laboratory equipment, microscopes, slides and pressure sterilizers. Kitasato would have presided, giving an impression of severe disapproval: steel-rimmed spectacles, downturned moustache, protruding lower lip that, when used judiciously, could convey such withering contempt. At his side were two highly qualified and eager deputies – Professor Tanemichi Aoyama and Dr Tohiu Ishigama – as well as three experienced assistants.

Yersin's departure for the plague slums of Hong Kong was a good deal less stately. Where Kitasato was setting off under presidential decree, Yersin's progress in Vietnam was stuttering and uncertain, frustrated at every turn by bureaucratic disagreement, misinformation and obfuscation. Yet, since his last stay in Saigon, there had been one welcome change in the colonial hierarchy: the Governor-General, Jean-Marie de Lanessan, had been replaced and his successor, Laurent Chavassieux, seemed to be a man who shared none of his predecessor's taste for wilful obstruction.

Yersin arrived in Saigon from the mountains on 17 May, and learned immediately – since the French would have been talking of little else – that just ten days before plague had made the leap from China to Hong Kong. Clearly, with the breaching of the defences of such a vital international port, his old petition – to study plague at its Yunnan frontier – was now obsolete, and a new plan was needed. In his memoir of those plague months he wrote – labouring over the sentences in his precise schoolbook hand, with its looping ascenders and perfectly balanced ballooning 'f's: 'The first thing I shall have to do in the study of plague is to look for its microbe; it is now evident that an initial microbiological study on plague will be much easier in Hong Kong than in Yunnan.'

With scarcely a break to debrief his expedition team or take a shower after the hard hike out of the jungle, Yersin hurried to the Governor's official residence. No doubt he'd have still been rehearsing his revised pitch to Chavassieux when he arrived at the sentried gates, only to be informed that the Governor had just left for a tour up-country. Yersin, undeterred, 'convinced M. Chavassieux will see things in the same light', set off in pursuit.

Some two weeks later in Qui Nonh, a fishermen's village on the way north to Hanoi, Yersin finally managed to track down Chavassieux. This is Vietnam's magnificent, and still largely unspoiled, tropical east coast; and here Yersin, on the pale-sand square of the village, the ground littered with shredded coconut husks, surrounded by a wall of curious faces, was at last able to put to effect all the arguments he'd spent so long reviewing. Chavassieux's answer was frustratingly equivocal: while he professed to see the merit in Yersin's argument, he refused to send him to Hong Kong without confirmation from Paris. Furthermore, he would take no decision until he had heard the latest from Yunnan. So go to Hanoi, he ordered Yersin: await orders there.

In Hanoi, on 3 June, Yersin's predicament was further complicated. In the hope of securing himself allies, he headed straight for the main hospital: with no appointment, he'd have marched directly to the suite of offices belonging to the chief of operations for 'health services' for the entire Indochinese colony. This man – referred to by Yersin simply as 'Trucy' – knew Yersin well, and would have had a good idea of the explorer-scientist's capabilities and enthusiasms; after hearing Yersin out, he agreed to send a telegram to Paris supporting his bid to go to Hong Kong. The response was immediate and forthright: orders remained unchanged;

a plague researcher was required in Yunnan, not Hong Kong, a job Chavassieux had earmarked for Yersin. As a colonial service doctor, he had no choice but to leave at once. No further delays would be tolerated.

Yet still Yersin hesitated, pondering his next move. If his experience of bureaucracy had taught him anything, it was to trust only in his own judgement, never to give quarter, and the more he learned of the instructions to leave for Yunnan, the more he determined to do all in his power to avoid it. Six days into his stay in Hanoi, the orders from high command in Paris still looming, he wrote to his mother that not only did Yunnan currently contain 'only a few isolated cases of plague', but it was also home, comically, to 'a colonel who fears the epidemic more than bullets, and who would like me to go there to attend him . . . which does not enter my mission at all.'

So Yersin, having no wish to end up as personal physician to a hypochondriac army officer, signed off his letter to his mother and began a telegram to his friend Albert Calmette, a Pasteur Institute-trained scientist now working in the health department at the colonial office. Calmette, who'd later go on to pioneer a tuberculosis vaccine, was Yersin's contemporary and also one of the few men with whom he felt properly relaxed. Yersin outlined the crisis, concluding by asking Calmette to appeal direct to the Foreign Ministry over the heads of the colonial authorities in Hanoi. This was his last chance, and he knew it.

On 9 June, a messenger arrived breathless at Yersin's Hanoi hotel. Yersin forced his thumb under the envelope flap, and tore open the seal. The enclosed was brief, succinct. Calmette had prevailed: Paris had finally backed

down. Yersin, as the Pasteur Institute's official researcher,
would be going to Hong Kong after all.

The bureaucratic manoeuvrings of the last three weeks
had cost Yersin vital laboratory time in Hong Kong, where
plague was now claiming at least a hundred new cases a
day. As time went on, research was becoming increasingly
hazardous. It was as well that Yersin, for the moment,
remained ignorant of the other major threat to his work: the
presence of a sizeable, well-connected and fully equipped
Japanese plague team which, by the time Yersin finally set
sail eastward three days later, was already disembarking at
Hong Kong harbour.

Chapter Five

IT WAS ONLY WHEN he woke to the sound of the telephone that he knew he'd been sleeping at all. The night was hot and windless; even with all the windows of the small apartment open there was no breeze, and he'd lain down naked beside his sleeping wife, slick with sweat.

After a while, lying there motionless, his newborn daughter snoring gently in the cot at the end of the bed, Mohanlal felt the heat become tolerable, but at this point, when he wanted sleep to come, he became aware of voices in the street below. He reached for his watch. One-thirty.

Noise at this hour was not unheard of, and on any other night he'd have rolled on his side and buried his head under the pillow. But this felt different: there was shouting, high-pitched argument, people clamouring to be heard. Across the road, he heard a window bang shut.

He swung his legs off the bed, walked to the window. From the balcony, under a sputtering orange streetlamp, he could make out a huddle of some thirty or so men. Despite the shrillness of the shouts, the palpable tension, this did not look like a brewing fight. There were hands on shoulders, wild gesticulations, a proximity that felt like brotherhood.

Puzzled, he stepped back inside. To block the noise he closed the windows behind him and, as compensation,

opened the front door instead. In the whitewashed stairwell
of the apartment block it was blessedly cool, and as he
made his way back to bed he hoped that he would finally
be able to sleep.

Yet he lay awake for what seemed hours, alive to his
wife's every murmur, to each catch in his little girl's
breathing. He heard the voices in the street fade, then
die. In a yard somewhere a dog began barking. Then the
telephone rang, breaking into a sleep he'd been certain
he'd never have, rousing him shakily from the bed.

'Yes?' His voice was barely a whisper.

'Don't drink the water. It's not safe.' A long pause. 'The
water.'

'Who is this?' He was suddenly awake. He looked across
at his still-sleeping wife, cupped a hand over the receiver.
'It's three in the morning.'

'Never mind that. Do as I say. The water is poisoned.'

'Why?' he whispered back, but even as he was speaking
he heard a click on the line, then the echo of his own voice,
loud in his ear.

He unplugged the phone and lay back on the bed, his
heart hammering. His wife had not stirred. Her forehead
was matt sheen; her pulse flickered in the hollow of her
neck, between the knuckles of her collarbones. He felt
himself merge with the bed, liquid with heat. He lay his
watch on his chest, no longer hoping for sleep, knowing
that before long his daughter would wake, crying to be fed.

When he heard the jangle of a telephone he was up
again, towel grabbed around him, before remembering that
of course his was now disconnected. He heard the ringing
tone twice more – the noise bright through the partition

wall – and then came old Banjeri's croaked hello. 'Water,' he kept saying, and then, louder, 'Do not . . . never again.'

'What . . . who's that?' His wife's voice, behind him, sounded blurred. He looked around. Her hand was raised to her face, but her eyes were still closed.

Across the stairwell he heard a door open. Mohanlal reached for his raincoat, threw the towel into a corner. He lifted the latch and closed the apartment door softly behind him.

'What's all this?' he called out to the other man, a diamond cutter who was coming out of his apartment hitching up his trousers, rubbing his eyes. 'What have you heard?'

'You had a telephone call?' The diamond cutter turned towards him, one hand on the stair rail.

'Yes. What is it? A practical joke?'

'The water. Is that what you heard?' They were close now, their voices lowered.

Mohanlal nodded. 'So you had it too. You believe it?'

The diamond cutter scratched his chin with a long fingernail, an audible stubble rasp. 'Who would do it? The Muslims? Not even they, I think.'

Interrupting them came the clunk of another apartment door. They turned to see Banjeri shuffle into the hallway. The gold weave of his slippers caught the light, glittered. He gave a tiny nod, barely acknowledgement, and stayed where he was, arms folded. Mohanlal and the diamond cutter, sensing deference was required, walked across to him.

'Mr Banjeri,' they said, in unison.

'I have lived too long,' the old man answered mournfully. 'When a man I do not know telephones me at three in the morning to tell me that poison now flows from my tap, then I would rather not be alive.'

The three men looked at each other in silence. Mohanlal was thinking of his wife: fearing her panic, he hoped she would sleep through, to wake in the morning to plausible explanations, the unmasking of some ineffectual hoaxer.

'We want to keep calm,' he said, as much to himself as the others. 'How could the water be poisoned? The whole city's water?'

'It is impossible,' Banjeri nodded, tugging a pendulous, liverish earlobe. 'I agree with you. But how to be sure?'

'I tell you who would know,' said the diamond cutter. 'Dr Shah. Mohanlal, you are a newspaper man: the doctor respects you. He does not listen to me. You go and ask him.'

Banjeri touched Mohanlal's shoulder. 'Good idea. Do it now.'

Mohanlal looked at his watch. Five-thirty. Behind other apartment doors he could hear early-morning noises: coughing, the gurgle of a plug. He gave a little bow and walked off down the passageway. He stopped at the fourth door, underneath an embossed gold nameplate: Dr Ramesh Shah, followed by a long string of letters. He pressed the doorbell. Nothing. He waited, then tried again. Still no response. He put his ear to the wood, but all he could hear was the muffled echo of other early risers, too indistinct to be coming from the doctor's apartment. Then suddenly, and with shocking force, he found himself banging his fist against the door. All around the stairwell doors opened.

'Come out, Shah,' Mohanlal shouted. 'Out of there.'

His neighbours were staring at him, men and women with sleep-tangled hair and bathrobes. He knelt down, put an eye to the letter box. Inside, a strip of light fell sideways across the passageway; the floor was strewn with books and clothes; the bed was stripped clean of sheets.

He stood up. His wife was standing at the doorway to their apartment, the baby against her shoulder. 'Mohanlal,' she began, but he raised a hand.

'Everybody, listen. The doctor is gone. Why has he gone? Since when did he ever go anywhere? I do not like it. Something bad is happening.'

*

IN THE CITY OF SURAT – a sprawl of diamond plants and textile factories, of squalor remarkable even by Indian standards – the summer of 1994 had been extreme. First the heat, then near three months of rain, July through to September, which saw the caramel-brown Tapti breach its banks and roll through most of town, forcing families on to their rooftops with what possessions they could salvage. When the floodwaters drew back, there was no white dove, no olive branch, just the sweet stench of decay: in every street bloated and split-open cows, dogs with sausage-fat, swollen tongues, goats with flies feasting on every blackened and distended orifice.

By the third week of September the floodwaters had mostly receded, leaving the streets ankle-deep in coagulant ooze. Householders tentatively climbed down from their rooftops, negotiating uncertainly through the slime that had once been their living-room floors. Worst hit was the working-class neighbourhood at the north end of the city – an area of low-built, rough concrete houses known as Ved Road after the north–south artery through its clogged heart – and here, on Wednesday 21 September, a young man and woman mysteriously collapsed and died within hours of each other. Their symptoms were identical – high fever, vomiting, breathlessness – but, in both cases, death had come too swiftly for a second medical opinion to be sought. Puzzled and not a little unnerved, none of the general practitioners who attended them attempted diagnosis.

By the evening, eight people were registered suddenly dead, although speculation – stoked by whispers and frenetic muttered confidences – had pumped this figure to nearer one hundred. To every death – both real and reported – there was a common theme: the afflicted were all young, or at least in early middle age, struck down 'in their prime'. By seven that evening, there was a growing crowd outside the New Civil Hospital, the city's largest. Wards were close to capacity, the wail of ambulance sirens was audible across town. In the main lobby – a huge concrete-pillared con-course, with rusty splashes of betel phlegm along the bottom of every wall – crowds were fighting to get to the drug counters. On the balcony above, a line of doctors scanned the mêlée: dressed head to toe in white, their faces masked, only their dark eyes visible.

*

THE GOVERNMENT-FUNDED New Civil Hospital was then, and remained, a bleakly ugly and unpromising forum for medicine. Built in 1972 from poured concrete – now chipped and crumbling – it sprawled across five or six acres of burnt-red, rubbish-strewn wasteland. The design seemed ill-thought-out and confusing, with related departments often a ten-minute walk from each other, along endless elevated walkways, past beggar women and their sad-eyed, ragged children. There were seven hundred and fifty beds

here, roughly half of which – outside an epidemic season –
lay empty, testament above all to the patients' parlous
recovery rate: the ratio of deaths to admissions, according
to the hospital's own figures, had been on the rise since
1981. No one out of choice, however grave his condition,
would allow himself to be transferred here; but treatment
was free, and most could not afford a private hospital.

The lifts were broken, desks piled high with sheaves of
yellowing paper. Outside, the scorched grass was littered
with vast lumps of concrete that were embedded in the
ground at strange angles, as if they'd fallen from the sky.

The official in charge was Dr Shailendra Vajpeyee, the
hospital's medical superintendent. He was a big man, heftily
built, hair brilliantined to a glossy black. September 1994,
he said, his smile dropping away, was 'unforgettable, the
experience of a lifetime'. On Monday 19 September, three
patients, all malaria suspects, were admitted into hospital;
two died before the night was out. By Wednesday morning,
senior doctors were muttering about pneumonia, and the
third patient, his breathing becoming harsher and more
erratic, was stretchered at a run to the X-ray room, where
pneumonia was duly diagnosed and treatment begun. That
afternoon, another patient was admitted – symptoms identical, the same breathlessness, high fever, sputum-filled cough
– and prescribed the same drug regimen. When neither
responded, something close to panic set in.

'Within hours,' Vajpeyee said, 'eight or nine patients
died, and if that was not bad enough, no one had any
idea of the cause.' An emergency meeting was called. The
hospital's most senior doctors, surgeons and administrators
argued furiously. It was dengue fever, insisted one; a mutant
strain of malaria, claimed another. A third carried news

from a nearby charitable hospital, where two more people
had died, both with the same symptoms. Finally, into a
room suddenly silent, one of the doctors spoke softly, with
certainty.

'The plague.'

Vajpeyee shrugged. 'What did we know? Only that a
large number of people had died in a very short time. That
we probably were witnessing the tip of an epidemic. So
what could it be? There is a rule of thumb: always suspect
the worst, the most dangerous disease – and there is none
more dangerous than plague.'

The mention of plague had thrown the room into
turmoil. Doctors fought to be heard. Wasn't plague a disease
of the past? Imagine the damage to India's reputation if it
had in fact resurfaced. Wasn't it possible, posited the head
of the medicine department, struggling to control his floun-
dering subordinates, that an outbreak had been triggered
by an earthquake the year before in the neighbouring state
of Maharashtra? The link between geological disturbance
and plague, he went on, was well known: rats die, their
plague-infected parasite fleas look for new hosts and end
up, as often as not, on the closest available human beings.
When this explanation met with silence, he ordered his
doctors to the hospital library. 'Read the textbooks,' he
barked.

The plague textbooks were hard to find, wedged behind
more recent publications on Aids, malaria, tuberculosis.
Two were unearthed, one twelve years old, the other twenty-
two: both were blotched with insect excreta; when cracked
open, the pages coughed dust. The volumes were forced
flat, indexes thumbed for 'clinical features'. Both texts
differentiated pneumonic from bubonic plague. Pneumonic

plague, the quicker-acting and more swiftly fatal, was marked by 'a chill, followed by fever, cough, and splinting of the chest, with the production of the sputum that soon becomes bloody . . . Progress of the disease is rapid, with extensive lung consolidation, septicaemia, prostration, mental confusion, subcutaneous haemorrhages due to intra-vascular coagulation, and shock, with death ensuing in two or three days.' The advice was unequivocal: treatment – large doses of the antibiotic tetracycline – should begin immediately.

For the hospital management this was proof enough: from this moment on, doctors were ordered, anything resembling pneumonia would be treated as plague. The doctors returned to their offices and wards sombrely, in silence. Warned of the dangers of contagion, they raided the stores for surgical masks; when supplies ran out, they covered their mouths and noses with handkerchiefs. Those with access to operating theatres stole in for surgical gloves; all covered their heads, leaving only the narrowest slits for eyes. By midnight on 21 September, twenty-five new patients had been admitted; seventy-two hours later, there would be more than four hundred.

By the next morning, with Surat's morning newspapers claiming a death toll of between three and four hundred, figures repeated unquestioningly by the BBC World Service, all normal life in the city had ceased. Shops remained shut; street vendors' pitches stayed empty. Buses out of town were loaded beyond capacity with families: women and children wedged inside, men on the roof. At the railway station fights broke out on the concourse as people tried to force themselves inside carriages already solid with refugees; women covered their mouths with folds of sari, the men with any rag that came to hand. There were vehicles of all kinds on the roads – pickups, scooters, Bajaj rickshaw taxis, goods trucks – but nothing was moving. Amid bleating horns, the dust and heat and desperation rose thick; the air was metallic, sour.

At the hospital, soldiers were posted outside the plague wards: two patients had already attempted escape. The militia were under orders to use force, and carried automatic rifles and full clips of shells. The outbreak, Vajpeyee admitted, caught the hospital completely unprepared: most years, the run of infectious diseases was at least predictable – plague, or so they'd imagined, had died out a generation ago.

'So we had to go on what we had heard, what we had read,' he said, clasping and unclasping his hands. 'For no one had seen the disease itself. All I could remember was that it killed ten, thirteen million people here in India between 1896 and some time in the 1930s. Before antibiotics, of course. That even a small epidemic could wipe out several hundred.'

The hospital, he said, designated by now the official plague centre, resorted to ferocious regimens of antibiotics – streptomycin, tetracycline, chloramphenicol – injected and in capsules, aware that pneumonic plague acted fast. 'If you get treatment within six hours,' Vajpeyee said, 'then most likely you can save the patient. After twelve hours, chances are fifty-fifty. After twenty-four hours, the outlook is very bleak.' So, as fast as surplus drugs came available, they were trucked to pharmacists across the city, and distributed door-to-door by a whole army of the white-coated and masked, bearing handfuls of miracle dust, whose mechanism was to most a mystery, that none the less accepted and consumed on faith.

During those first days he slept little. Whenever he returned home from the hospital, his telephone would be ringing. 'Friends, anybody who knew me, they all called me on the telephone. They wanted to know if they should stay in the city. I told them that nobody could guarantee that they would be safe either if they left or if they stayed. "Look at me," I told them. "I am working here with my patients. I am staying. If you want to leave us, well, that is up to you." ' Of all his acquaintances, he nodded, allowing himself a quiet smile, not one joined the half-million-strong exodus from the city.

'But,' he added, 'I do not wish to give the wrong impression. There is a side to this story that gives me no pride at all. On those first days, when the panic in the city was very large, and many thousands were fleeing, people tried to go to their family doctors for help. These are private practitioners, you understand, and they have clinics on every street corner, but when their patients needed them, they were not there: all such clinics were closed. Why? Because the doctors had been the first to flee, driving far from town as soon as they heard that plague had broken out. And I ask you: what were the people to think then?'

Chapter Six

IT SITS BECALMED, its reflection a dark shadow on the still water. It fills most of the frame, though the rough grain of the print and the lack of sharp detail make one suspect that the photograph was once part of a broader shot, cropped for focus. It is a vessel, but one unlike any other. In harsh and geometric monochrome, it appears forbidding, almost predatory. There is no fore- or afterdeck, just a straight-line vertical – blinding white, of wood or plate metal – from gunwale to roof gutter. Into these walls are cut windows of varying shapes and sizes, but all black and featureless, with no visible frames or glass. Near bow and stern the windows are wider, squatter; amidships they shrink to arrow-slits, close together. The roof is pitched, with fifteen or so stovepipe chimneys. There is a flagpole, but no flag. With the dark mountains behind, the ship appears ghostly and alone. It would, one cannot help thinking, make an excellent penitentiary, reserved for the most determined and malign recidivists.

Little wonder, then, that this malevolent-looking hulk, pressed into service at the start of May 1894 as a floating plague hospital, should have become an object of terror. Moored some three hundred yards off the Hong Kong waterfront, *Hygeia* – a name redolent more of wishful thinking than any proven curative powers – was immediately designated a dedicated treatment centre for plague-stricken Chinese. This was straightforward racial segregation, however vigorously Dr James Lowson, superintendent of the Government Civil Hospital, tried to justify it on medical grounds. Lowson argued against allowing the Chinese to be treated in their own hospital, the Tung Wah, claiming that it would be impossible to prevent contagion spreading into the community. Far safer for everyone, he told the assembled doctors and colonial officials at the 11 May extraordinary meeting of the sanitary committee, for the diseased to be out of sight, offshore, from where there would be no escape.

As *Hygeia* filled up with the moaning and feverish and dying – and not one Chinese doctor accepted Lowson's 'invitation' to inspect the facilities and conditions on board – opposition hardened into something darker, more indicative of the underlying hatred the Chinese had always felt for their colonial masters. In front of the busy streets of Hong Kong, like a lone actor on the stage of a packed amphitheatre, lay the *Hygeia* – a constant reminder of all that was unequal and unjust about this two-tier society. As they stared from their tenements and back alleys out across the water to the spectral white hulk, the Chinese began to tell each other that something far worse than medicine was being practised by the European doctors on board, those men in white coats whose masked faces would occasionally flash into focus at the windows, then slink into darkness again.

Most insistent of all such rumours was the first story to gain currency: that *Hygeia* was a hospital in name only, and was shortly to become a sinister form of laboratory, with the end product a 'new and certain cure for the plague', the raw materials for which were the livers of Chinese children. Anticipating a military-swift conscription of schoolchildren, mothers withdrew their offspring from classes: by mid-May, more than half the Chinese schools, bereft of pupils, were closed. Other fantasists claimed that an industrial-scale infanticide was planned, with the government aiming to bury alive some twenty thousand babies, although no reason for such barbarism was ever given.

Feeling themselves cornered and overpowered, the Chinese began their own form of disease prevention, which involved long and raucous street processions, headed by the portered likeness of a Chinese deity, and accompanied by the machine-gun rattle of firecrackers. In this atmosphere of mutual suspicion it took little to stoke the flames of paranoia, and newspaper reporters, true to type, did their bit. 'Is it a fact,' enquired a 'correspondent' of the *Hong Kong Telegraph*, 'that a Chinese woman was sent on board the *Hygeia* by the Sanitary Authorities supposed to be suffering from the plague, but which proved to be a case of pregnancy? And is it true that the mistake was not found out until it was too late to save the patient's life?'

It was not long before every gesture of the colonial government in the direction of hygiene was greeted with clamorous animosity by the Chinese. The efforts of the three hundred volunteers from the Shropshire Light Infantry to act as plague monitors, inspecting houses in the most crowded Chinese quarters, incited violent clashes. By 21 May, one of the accompanying sanitary inspectors had even gone so far as to plead his case before the magistrates' court: attempting to enter a house, he had been driven back by a mob hurling rocks and bricks. The accused – three housewives – were found guilty and fined.

Even on the rare occasions when the soldiers' work progressed smoothly – when the targeted house turned out to be abandoned, the inhabitants having fled north into China – it was repulsive, gruelling labour. They'd rise at dawn, then head out from barracks at seven thirty, armed with buckets and limewash, trailed by a reluctant posse of press-ganged 'coolies'. They'd start on the ground floor, scrubbing furniture, clothing, scouring pots and frying pans, then move upstairs. According to an anonymous witness, the decrepitude beggared description, and tested to the full the vocabulary of disgust. 'All paper was torn off the walls and woodwork, and then, in all its nakedness, you saw the filth of these dwellings. Vermin of all sorts were found crawling everywhere, and heaps of rubbish and filth lay disregarded in odd corners . . . Water was brought in buckets from the cookhouse, and a commencement was made of getting the floor clean. It is impossible to give any conception of the filth which was then swept down the stairs – it must have been seen to be believed.'

News of British soldiers kicking down doors in the Chinese quarters of Hong Kong, hurling furniture into the street and slooshing the furniture with acrid detergent spread quickly to Canton, the closest mainland Chinese city and the one from which most Hong Kong Chinese families originated. Within days, a slew of posters had gone up all over the city, warning that the entire European population faced massacre should anyone dare condemn Cantonese dwellings on grounds of health. To compound this, word was put about that the despised foreigners were also distributing poisoned scent bags. No European felt safe; two female missionaries, guilty of nothing more than attempting to stretcher a plague victim to hospital, were hounded and stoned.

Chinese leaders in Hong Kong, fearing army reprisals, opted in the end for opposition of an altogether more decorous, fittingly British, nature. On 22 May, a delegation arrived on foot at the great porticoed entrance to Government House with a written petition containing four demands: an end to the enforced military inspection of their houses; that plague sufferers might be allowed free passage home to Canton; that those remaining be treated exclusively in the Tung Wah, their own hospital; and that, henceforth, the funereal hulk *Hygeia* be no longer an epidemic hospital for the Chinese.

Most Chinese no doubt regarded the petition as a ludicrous piece of window-dressing, not least the clause requesting unhindered return to Canton. For, throughout May, Chinese from all over the colony – permission or no – had been fleeing in their thousands. Official figures, tallied at quayside, listed 76,036 people having quit Hong Kong that month, with only 42,390 arrivals – a shortfall of more than thirty-three thousand. As May became June, the graph rose ever faster, forcing construction work and manufacturing, shipping and food production to a point near closedown. The Hong Kong Rope Works shut its doors, dismissing its few remaining staff, as did the Lee Yuen Sugar Refinery. Mail boats, fearful of touching land, tethered postal bags to buoys, turning for the open sea before the pickup launch was even within hailing distance. By the beginning of June, this once-bustling harbour lay abandoned, the only figures on the dock the white-uniformed soldiers, the only water traffic the solitary, low-slung coffin barge on its continual passage to and from the burial pits.

Within two weeks of the start of the epidemic, the main hospitals – the Europeans' Government Civil Hospital, under Lowson, and the Chinese community's Tung Wah – reached capacity. Backing down under pressure from the Chinese, the government pledged to cease sending Chinese plague patients to the *Hygeia*, and instead pressed into service an arguably far more pestilential venue, an abandoned glass factory in Kennedy Town, whose only conceivable merit was its proximity to the burial pits. First-hand accounts make it clear that this was not a building in which any man would have willingly chosen to spend his time. Lowson's diary entry for 24 May contains a retrospective scribble, and despite the passage of some four decades, he remembers scenes that 'baffled description. When I think of it now [1933], I wonder how anyone came out of it alive.'

A photograph from one of the first days of the factory's life as a plague hospital shows a long room with bare floorboards, just wide enough to allow a walkway between two rows of bodies. Some thirty men are visible, lying on their backs on reed mats. Their heads are turned towards the photographer, eyes glassy, cheeks sunken. They are covered in a variety of rags and army-issue blankets. It must have been hot – this was the eve of monsoon, and the windows along both walls are thrown open – yet the patients, icy with rising fever, clutch their clothing around them. Men lie on their sides, hands between legs for warmth. Nowhere is there any sign of medicine, nor any doctor.

The comparison between the derelict glass factory, designated Chinese-only, and the other temporary hospital – set up on 14 May in Kennedy Town police station for afflicted Europeans as well as those Chinese willing to

submit to Western medicine – could not have been starker.
Both were in the same neighbourhood, but there any simi-
larity ended. The police station, according to one source,
was 'surrounded by a wide verandah, open on all sides,
[and] is admirably suited to the purpose. Everything and
everywhere is clean, bright and cheerful. The officer in
charge is radiant, and the sisters from the Civil Hospital,
who take turns at this work, are the embodiment of kind
activity and considerate attention.' There was no shortage
of bedding, food and medicine, and all the patients appeared
optimistic of recovery. The glass factory, by contrast, was
'decayed and ruinous', filled with 'moribund' patients, all
of whom 'seemed occupied with dying'. Overcrowding was
so severe that patients lay half on top of one another,
'impatiently resenting the overlapping hand or foot of the
next neighbour'. There was no sign of food, 'either adminis-
tered or in preparation'. When night came, the sick silently
covered their faces with their blankets, a motion that spoke
most eloquently of despair, of the fact that few expected to
see dawn.

As the death toll continued to rise, so the white population did its best to remain aloof. Thus far, after all, plague
had confined itself to the 'native classes' – clear testament
to the causal link between moral decay and disease.
However, while on one level reassuring, the racial bias of
the contagion had one lamentable side-effect for the colonial
classes. 'The scare among the Chinese was spreading to the
private coolies and house "boys",' one witness complained.
'Many left without giving any warning, and Europeans
began to fear they would find themselves without servants.'
Even wealth – of which there was no more certain marker
than a mansion on the prestigious, airy upper slopes of

Victoria Peak – was no protection against the loss of staff, for a new rumour had caught alight among the Chinese that the plague had been caused not by 'filth', as the Europeans kept insisting, but by the methods of construction of the Peak Railway, the funicular tramline that cut straight from the heart of the business district to the summit of Victoria Peak, 1,825 feet above. The rails, it was claimed, had not been lain on traditional wooden sleepers but upon the yielding bodies of Chinese babies: plague was the gods' inevitable punishment for such wickedness.

Yet a far bleaker scenario now lay in prospect for the colonial classes. 'Soon,' flailed an editorial in the *Hong Kong Telegraph*, 'every European will have to wash his own shirt and pull his own rickshaw!' And it would have been with just this kind of doomsday in mind that the worshippers gathered at St John's Cathedral on Sunday 3 June to hear a special prayer of deliverance from plague, and to ruminate on the Reverend R. F. Cobbold's sermon on Ezekiel 8: 19 – 'For I have no pleasure in the death of him that dieth, said the Lord God; wherefore turn yourselves and live ye.'

Unbeknown to Cobbold and his packed and uncommonly prayerful congregation, however, the first two white men to contract plague were at that very moment breathing their last in the sepulchral gloom of the *Hygeia*, their final memory of the fading world the clank-clank of the anchor chain and the whisper, like the spirits of the world to come, of the harbour swell against the hull.

*

To those blessed with the gift of retrospective wisdom, plague came as no great surprise. To some Chinese, it was necessary to look no further than the forests where, for the first time in thirty years, the bamboo had flowered prodigiously: a certain omen of ill. To the Europeans, who'd have scorned such a belief as wayward superstition, the roots of the disease were more various, though scarcely more accurate or scientific.

Dr Alexander Rennie, consular surgeon for Canton and the first white man to report on the epidemic, proposed that plague was triggered by contaminated and insufficient water, poor ventilation, but above all by 'filth'. As reassurance to his readers, he dismissed any notion that it might be contagious, certainly outside the crowded Chinese neighbourhoods. This theory was expanded by Governor Sir William Robinson, who added the bold and entirely unsubstantiated coda that it was the recent drought which had caused the outbreak, since the consequent depletion of reservoirs had meant less water for cleaning streets, drains and houses. Dr James Lowson was broadly of the same opinion, although he – like Rennie, emphasizing the causal role of 'poverty and dirt' – credited a few days of heavy rain with the ability to flush out the 'poison . . . [which] is not infectious or contagious'. Others, like Royal Navy surgeon Herbert Penny, were less sure as to plague's contagiousness: most likely, he contended, the disease was carried in clothing, and transmitted through contact.

In non-scientific circles – in these weeks before the arrival of Yersin and Kitasato – opinions were no less erratic. Within days of the first case, the correspondence columns of the newspapers filled with a clamour of competing theories, all equally convinced of their own validity, all equally wayward. Tobacco, wrote one reader, was a 'simple preventative', and should be made freely available to all soldiers – a claim that at least had its historical precedent: chewing tobacco leaves was used in Stuart times as a plague prophylactic, and Pepys wrote in his diary that, during the 1665 London plague, 'an ill conception of myself and my smell . . . forced [me] to buy some roll tobacco to smell and chaw, which took away the apprehension.' So efficacious was the weed held to be that, in times of plague, even schoolchildren were forced to partake: an Eton schoolboy is recorded as being 'never whipped so much in his life as he was one morning for not smoking'.

While there was no propagandist in Hong Kong who would have dared suggest such an extreme punishment for refusing to inhale, there was a consensus in favour of an approach that was altogether more wanton. Taipingshan, the overcrowded Chinese district at the centre of the epidemic, should be demolished; better still, wrote one newspaper correspondent in the first week of June, burned to the ground. 'It is quite clear the poisonous gas issues from certain particular localities . . . the only sure measure to stamp out plague is to burn down infected houses.'

'Sir,' countered another voice, 'it is rumoured that Taipingshan is to be utterly demolished. *Cui bono?* Such a measure would have as much effect in curing or even preventing the plague as whitewashing the walls; that is, none whatever. It isn't in the walls, nor yet in the bricks. It is in the filth-saturated soil,' a state of affairs he laid unequivocally at the government's door for introducing a drainage system 'which not one in thirty of the population for generations to come but will abuse; that is, as soon as the pipes are laid they proceed to choke or break them and consequently the soil gets saturated.'

The signs – the proliferation of ever-wilder theories, their misplaced rage and whiff of recrimination – pointed to a community under siege. All that was needed now was a scapegoat, and the Europeans were of one voice: immigrants. Plague, hollered the press, was 'due to the vast influx of the filthy mendicants and coolies . . . imagine this lot all huddled together . . . reeking with filth, many of them diseased.' The only solution – propounded in language beloved of xenophobic despots down the ages – was to 'purify' the island by expelling the infected.

As this racist rhetoric was reaching its shrill climax, two foreign scientists – Professor Shibasaburo Kitasato and Dr Alexandre Yersin – disembarked in Hong Kong harbour within three days of each other, stepping straight into an atmosphere so charged with distrust and venom it might have been wartime.

Chapter Seven

WHEN PROFESSOR KITASATO and his entourage arrived in Hong Kong on 12 June 1894, the news would have been conveyed in a frenzied instant, an electric tremor of excited voices spreading word of hope, that plague had at last found a proper adversary: this disembarking foreigner, whispered the fearful, was their saviour. In houses up the mountainside – from the customs house to the mansions in the shadow of the peak – people unbolted their shutters and risked an inrush of infectious air on the chance of a snatched glimpse of the sober-suited, reputedly brilliant, Japanese bacteriologist.

Had luck been with them, they would have seen a rare commotion at the quayside, the arrival of a boat with noticeably foreign lines and markings, porters busy on deck as they handed ashore a line of dark leather trunks, suitcases, boxes. Such activity would have been instantly remarkable: the last month had seen total shutdown of port traffic, as shipping lines from across the world diverted their vessels from Hong Kong. Compared to the sporadic and lethargic motion of the floating hearse on its way to and from the burial pits, the bustle and industry of Kitasato's arrival would have seemed thrilling, an occasion of consequence.

Kitasato stepped on to the jetty in his customary white suit, accompanied by five others, looking like a posse of tropical undertakers. It had taken them seven days to make the crossing from Tokyo, and all the way, barely sleeping, they'd have chewed over possible theories and lines of attack. Kitasato – dominant, confident, brooding – would have presided, incontestably the expedition leader, already, back home, the grand scientific hero. As to the intricacies of his character, there are fewer clues: he published sparingly and, unlike Yersin, kept his rages and passions to himself: no diary or letters survive in the public domain.

From his published papers and speeches comes a sense of an austere professional, secure in his methodology and diagnoses, whose interest in the culture of Chinese Hong Kong into which the plague had suddenly thrown him was proscribed and over-simplified, perhaps plain uninterested. Unlike Yersin – whose reaction to the lives of the Chinese, in all their undisguised squalor and otherness, was breathless, both fascinated and horrified – Kitasato responded to what he saw with economy and detachment. Speaking to the Private Hygiene Society of Japan at the end of 1894, he compressed six or so weeks of observation into a hundred words of blunt description. Chinese houses, he instructed his audience, were 'constructed on the top of each other, with box-like rooms that are generally very small, without sunshine. I wonder why they do not live in larger rooms.'

Kitasato was pragmatic, private, fiercely competitive. He arrived in Hong Kong confident of victory, that the prize of plague was within his grasp. He'd taken no chances: his backup team was of the highest calibre: among the other five was the renowned pathologist Professor Tanemichi Aoyama from the Tokyo Medical School, a top government official, and bacteriologist Dr Tohiu Ishigama, seconded as Kitasato's chief assistant.

With their surgical instruments, trunks of clothes and pressure sterilizers unloaded and secured to a trap, Kitasato ordered a fleet of rickshaws to carry him and his team to the residence of the Japanese consul. Here, in pale-columned splendour, served green tea by deferential Chinese footmen, Kitasato would have allowed himself a modest smile of satisfaction as the Consul expressed, in the laboured and minutely formal Japanese fashion, the extent of the Emperor's, and the colony's, pleasure at his safe arrival. One can picture him – his appearance assembled from the handful of portraits that survive – as resolute and inscrutable despite travel fatigue, his moustache maybe a little bushier than the usual tight crop, those small eyes behind the circular steel-rimmed spectacles darker, more tired.

Before long, Kitasato would install his team in the Hong Kong Hotel, but for his first night at least, he probably looked no further than the guest suites of the Consul's official residence. It would have been rare for the Consul to have had the honour of extending hospitality to visitors, certainly ones this eminent and propitious. So he would have been expecting them to stay under his roof, their rooms and sleeping mats already prepared, flowers arranged in welcome, praying silently that they had not already had a better offer: from the Governor himself, say, whose invitation would have been impossible to turn down. While his guests began to unpack their cases, to wash and shave in anticipation of the combat to come, the Consul – against the backdrop of a flaring orange sunset, a sight that spoke to him now not of beauty but of corruption and disease – would have proudly dispatched his messenger with the news that Kitasato had arrived. The great man – long and excitedly awaited – was finally here.

All through that first night – as on most summer nights in Hong Kong then and now – the rain would have hammered on the groove-tiled roofs of the colony's villas and tenements, its shanties and hospitals. June is the island's hottest and wettest month, with rainfall during those four weeks regularly topping sixteen inches, and temperatures well into the thirties. In 1894, the monsoon started early; before the end of May, soldiers on cleanup parties were often seen in full waterproofs – oilskins and sou'westers – hurrying under cover with each new cloudburst, the strength of the downpour detonating a knee-level haze. On 28 May the temperature reached such a pitch that, in the temporary hospital in the derelict glass factory, windows were left permanently open, and from those whose hinges were too seized to move, the glass was punched clear.

*

EARLY THE NEXT MORNING, 13 June, Kitasato led his team to a fleet of waiting rickshaws and – in his punctilious but limited English – ordered the drivers to take them to the Government Civil Hospital, where he was scheduled to meet Dr James Lowson. With the monsoon exploding suddenly to life again, he pulled his raincoat tight about him, lifting his patent leather shoes from the rising pool of water in the footwell. He'd have become quickly confused, too, disoriented by the endless switchbacks as the rickshaws struggled up the incline. After a while, the view was of roofs – the cramped back-to-backs of Taipingshan – then the harbour beyond, looking less than turquoise now through the blear of rain. Finally, at an elevation of some generosity and airiness, there appeared the grand vista of the Government Civil Hospital itself, classical in ambition and design, fronted by a gracious, curving driveway, distinguished architecturally by the vaulted colonnade through which, as the rain finally eased, a huddle of white-coated men now came running.

At their head was a tall, pale-skinned and moustachioed European, big bony hand outstretched. As he approached, Kitasato – climbing down from his rickshaw and beating the rainwater from his coat – noticed Lowson's distinguishing feature, a misaligned right eye that, veering wide, gave the impression that he was somehow not seeing you at all. In serious mood – as in formal photographs, straight-backed and sober – this effect was heightened, but now, as he bounded across the gravel, grinning broadly despite the tension and grief of the past few weeks, there was no mistaking the pleasure and relief as he greeted Kitasato and vigorously pumped his hand.

Later, in a report he wrote for the *Lancet*, Kitasato would publicly acknowledge his gratitude to Lowson, who 'put everything at our disposal in the most friendly spirit'. This was a magnificent understatement: Lowson in fact did everything but prostrate himself at Kitasato's feet; had he a cloak he would have lain it across the puddles that glittered now in the hospital driveway. For this Scottish medic, raised in the small east-coast town of Forfar, educated at the University of Edinburgh, and still only twenty-eight at the start of the plague epidemic, the chance to work alongside such an eminent figure would have, until now, seemed laughably remote. Certainly, like all ambitious young doctors, Lowson would have read of Kitasato's groundbreaking tuberculosis work and would no doubt have agreed with the *British*

Medical Journal's encomium that the Japanese scientist was, 'next to Koch, the greatest bacteriologist in the world'. Now that Kitasato was finally here, Lowson would have felt his own excitement building: if, as he now believed, Kitasato was destined to go down in history as the conqueror of plague, he, as Kitasato's right-hand man, would also be showered with glory.

Lowson outlined his plans. He had, he explained, reserved rooms in one of the temporary plague hospitals for use as Kitasato's laboratory and autopsy suite. He'd have put considerable effort into organizing this, determined that Kitasato should have the very best facilities in the cleanest of the hospitals. In the end he'd chosen the hospital set up in the Kennedy Town police station. Though never intended to be anything other than a police headquarters, the building – Lowson told Kitasato as they shared a rickshaw across town – made a superlative hospital.

Arriving for the first time, Kitasato would have been struck above all by the contrast between the hospital and the neighbourhood that surrounded it. From the central district of Victoria, with its whitewashed merchants' headquarters and spacious quayside offices, they'd passed through cramped and abandoned Taipingshan – the houses now boarded-up and shuttered, an occasional ghostly face at a high window, piles of rubbish smoking in the streets and side alleys – and on westward, the houses growing ever more ramshackle and part-roofed, rotting corpses lying in gutters, their unclothed limbs askew. By the time they reached the hospital, they were in a landscape almost entirely devoid of buildings, with the scrubby lower slopes of Mount Davis ahead of them, on which a group of men was at work. It looked like earthworks, some kind of construction.

Lowson leant towards Kitasato. 'Plague pits,' he explained. 'Gravediggers.'

As they began their tour of the hospital, Lowson would have done his best to concentrate on the positive: he'd have glossed over the conspicuous failure in medication, in particular his own doubtful concoction prescribed for all the plague hospitals, which consisted of beaten eggs, frothed milk, and an unspecified 'stimulant'. Instead, he'd have focused on the Kennedy Town hospital's supposed selling points: the abundance of fresh air; the 'hopeful and cheerful' patients, almost all Chinese, many of whom were said to be 'full of merriment'; the sufficiency of bedding, medicine and food; the overspill cots on a section of shady veranda; the availability of clean water, gas, even the use of a telephone. Yet, only one year on, sitting down to write his official plague report, Lowson – no longer anxious to impress any visiting dignitaries – spoke plainly of the site's shortcomings. Being close to Mount Davis may have provided convenient access to the plague pits, he said, but trees on the nearby slopes 'made [the hospital] a hunting ground for flies and mosquitoes which sometimes added greatly to our patients' sufferings'. He added sourly, 'The arrangements of the rooms also left much to be desired.'

Kitasato's first impressions, however, were highly favourable, and he ordered his team straightaway to begin unpacking his equipment – microscopes, slide trays, sets of scalpels and scissors, pressure sterilizers, surgical gloves and masks. Mirroring the layout of an established laboratory, he'd have set up tables along all walls, to form an extended workbench, leaving room in the middle for the dissection of corpses. All the while, hovering in the background, unable to conceal his boyish excitement, would have been Lowson, chattering to the professor's back, as the older man uncased his instruments and screwed together lenses, recounting the story so far: the wild rumours, the forced inspections of houses, the ensuing riots.

It had been, Lowson informed Kitasato – moving closer now, his voice lowering to a whisper – a terrible month, with Hong Kong as if under siege, the disease itself almost a bombardment, forcing people to hide away, fearful and suspicious, trusting no one. Chinese and Western doctors shared almost no common ground. When the European physicians insisted on isolating plague patients – preferably on the offshore hulk *Hygeia* – the Chinese told each other that the vessel, when full, was going to sail for Europe, where the bodies would be ground into powder and fed as prophylactic medicine to the continent's nobility. In their efforts to prevent this happening, they did everything they could to keep the rate of infection secret. The moment a military search party arrived in a street, corpses would be smuggled from house to house; on one occasion, with every exit barred, and the soldiers closing in, a plague corpse was propped up at a mah-jong game, eyes fixed strangely on the ceiling, claw hand outstretched, tiles in an untouched pile before it.

Of most pressing concern to Kitasato, however, was having unfettered access to corpses to conduct experiments, but he understood already that this would not be straight-forward: the Chinese – who did not believe that the cause of medicine was advanced by cutting open bodies – would not willingly countenance dismemberment of their dead. Lowson, who'd have sensed Kitasato's growing disquiet as his laboratory preparations neared their end, would have done his best to reassure him. There was a loophole, he explained, which would guarantee secrecy: according to hospital regulations, doctors were obliged to carry out post-mortems without consulting the family of the deceased. The rioting, the brick-throwing and stoning that this had already engendered would not, said Lowson, prevent post-mortems being attempted.

Kitasato – not a man to scare easily – suddenly felt frightened. In the text of a speech made shortly after his return home, a rare clue to his feelings survives. Detailing the obstacles to autopsy – the certain Chinese opposition, the gulf between the different cultural and medical approaches to contagion – he breathed deeply and told it straight: 'If the Chinese had found out about the post-mortem examinations, we would have been beaten to death on the spot.' Clearly, Lowson's placatory words, his assurances of round-the-clock guards and extra medical support, did little to set Kitasato's mind at peace.

So it would have been in darkly reflective mood that Kitasato led his team back that evening to the Hong Kong Hotel. No doubt Lowson – brooding alone as his rickshaw clattered over the cobbles after the convoy of Japanese – would have been longing to escort Kitasato back to his residence, to install him and his colleagues in the palatial but seldom-used guest wing, but Kitasato had been adamant: he did not wish to impose on Dr Lowson's kindness. Besides, Hong Kong, even under the rumble of incipient monsoon, made a thrilling destination for the traveller, even one as disinclined to the holiday spirit as Professor Shibasaburo Kitasato.

Before retiring for the night, it is not hard to picture

the solitary bacteriologist succumbing to the temptation to ride the elevator – the hotel's 'Hydraulic Ascending Room' – and, at the top of its climb, taking a few minutes to absorb the prospect before him. There was the harbour, black and deserted now, the palest shadow through the rain marking the position of the hospital hulk *Hygeia*; turning inland he could see the hills and city through which plague, even as he watched, was stalking malignant. As he stood there, full of imaginings and sudden plans, he would have felt a swelling in his chest, a sense that his arrival in Hong Kong at this moment was indeed – as Lowson had been breathlessly intoning all afternoon – the start of something epic and unforgettable. The red carpet had been laid out before him; all he had to do was take the first step.

Chapter Eight

MOHANLAL PUT AN ARM around his wife, guided her back into their apartment and closed the door. He knew that his neighbours would be wanting to speak to him, to probe further, as at previous moments of community tension, assuming that he as the newspaper man had access to some kind of privileged knowledge – but there were things, first, that he needed to discuss with his wife.

He tried to lead her to the table, but she pulled away from him; the baby began to cry, little yelping stabs that made it impossible to think, splintered his thoughts. He put a hand over his eyes.

'Couldn't you feed her?' His voice came out strained, reedy.

She sat on the edge of the bed and did as he said. The baby quietened and he felt the pressure in his head subside, but still his wife would not look at him.

'Hetal,' he pleaded. 'Are you trying to punish me? What have I done?'

'It is not you,' she mumbled, speaking so softly he had to kneel close to hear the words. 'I am frightened. What is going on?'

'I do not know, but look, I am going to find out.' He would get to the office, telephone her from there. 'And I will come back for lunch. We can talk then.'

He heard the noise of the street – the shouting and car horns, the angry whine of scooters – before he'd even reached the front door of the apartment block. Once outside, an astonishing sight greeted him: it was only six-thirty, but the road was impassable. At the corner, two buses were wedged nose-to-nose, the drivers shouting at each other through the windscreens. They were blocking the side-road, but there was no possibility of movement: behind each and on all sides were trucks, scooters, cars, jammed bumper-to-bumper. Only pedestrians appeared to be moving, and that uncertainly: Mohanlal saw a man and a woman climb on to the bonnet of an old Datsun, only to stop the moment they had done so, looking around, shaking their heads. Under the man's mask he could see he was shouting, the cotton gauze over his mouth wet, gathering dirt.

Normally, he'd have taken his scooter to work, but one look at the mêlée before him was enough to convince him to pocket his keys again and push through on foot. Elbows and shoulders jabbed and jostled him; the old-curry smell of sweat and panic assaulted his senses. Yet, in the midst of it, there was a sudden silence; the shouting fell away, and in the space he heard his own voice, rising over the dust and blue diesel.

'What is this? What is happening?'

Back came a chorus of voices. 'Plague. We're leaving this place. Everyone is dying.'

'Plague?' he yelled back, but all was clamour again. He pushed onward, more desperately now, aiming to reach the corner where he knew of a cut-through. He kept his head down, but felt himself crowded on all sides: black eyes, the ghostly white slashes of masks, hands clawing at his clothing. He clutched his briefcase to his chest: half shield, half battering ram.

At the corner, garbage was banked high in the entrance to the cut-through: a deliberate obstruction, he guessed. The stench, even so early in the morning, was foetid and vinegary but he launched himself up it anyway, feeling it yield underfoot, each handhold a sugary mash of banana skin and sodden cardboard, mouldering fruit husks and empty ant-infested tins. At the top, as ultimate deterrent, lay the skew-legged corpse of a mongrel pup, both eyes gone, bright red sockets swarming with flies. Looking away, covering his mouth, Mohanlal almost tripped. He reached the bottom at a run, skidding on some unseen ooze.

Then he ran, pelted from doorways with husks of bread and old fruit; from a top window an arc of dishwater caught him on the side of the face.

The newspaper office was besieged, angry fists demanding information, as if the reporters inside weren't already doing all they could. He pulled out his security pass, but as soon as he did so hands clawed at him, and he closed it tight in his fist again. Still some ten yards from the door, he shouted for the guard, hollering his name and forcing his way forward till the peaked cap with the gold portcullis turned towards him and the guard reached out a long arm over the heads of the crowd and pulled Mohanlal through.

It was scarcely calmer in the newsroom. Normally at this hour – ninety minutes or so from deadline for the afternoon edition – there was a quiet hubbub, the percussion of typewriter keys, the shouts of the copy boys. Today, though, all the reporters and sub-editors were gathered in a tight group in the middle of the room, the editor standing

on a chair, facing them. He looked up when he saw
Mohanlal.

'So you made it. We're just wrapping up. What have
you heard?'

'Plague, poisoned water, you name it.'

'It's plague, for sure,' said one of the junior reporters,
spooling through his notepad. 'You seen the morning
papers?'

The discussion became general, chaotic. The editor
stepped down from his chair and gestured to Mohanlal,
who pushed through the scrum. The older man crossed the
newsroom, entered the glass cubicle at the far end and
waited for Mohanlal to join him. Mohanlal closed the door
and took the proffered chair.

'Well,' the editor sighed, sinking heavily into his own
chair behind the desk. 'Have we all gone crazy?'

'I'm sorry?' Mohanlal answered. 'Crazy?'

'I had a call this morning from Vadilal − remember
him, he's on the *New York Times* now − and guess what he
said? That between three and four thousand have died in
Surat these last two days. On good authority, he said. It
was all I could do to make him hold off for a day. Where
does he get those figures?'

'There's a doctor who lives in my block,' Mohanlal said.
'I tried to get hold of him this morning, but he wasn't there.
This is the first time he's gone anywhere. That causes me
concern.'

'He's not the only one.' The editor's eye was twitching.
He pressed two fingers to the side of his face. 'We've been
getting reports all morning of doctors having fled. In
Katargam the people have burned down a doctor's surgery.

Smashed it to pieces, then threw a match into the petrol tank of his Bajaj.'

'What do they say down at the New Civil Hospital?' Mohanlal asked, barely hearing what the editor had said. He was beginning to feel excited, that old war-zone thrill. 'How many dead have they got down there?'

'It's plague, all right,' the editor said wearily. 'What do the morning papers say? Fifty? The hospital doesn't know any better than that.'

'But what about Vadilal? The New York figures?'

'That,' he said, leaning forward over his bank of telephones, the blotting pad and strewn pens, 'is what I want you to find out.'

Back at his desk, before even clearing the papers off his chair to sit down, Mohanlal telephoned home. He stood, receiver crooked in his shoulder, gazing numbly at the disorder that was his professional life – a half-eaten nan bread, an ashtray full of tea bags, a three-foot pile of old newspapers – and waited as the line crackled and clicked. It rang, then carried on ringing. He imagined his wife bathing the baby, or fixing a bottle. He knew she'd be there, since he'd made her promise to await his call. Yet it rang, and rang. Another reporter approached him, wanting a name and telephone number, and Mohanlal leafed through his contacts book, scribbled the number, then put the receiver to his ear again. It was still ringing. He held the phone at arm's length, as if it had some kind of animate nature of its own, as if perhaps it knew what was happening at the other end. Then, abruptly, he dropped it back in the cradle.

An hour later, headache building, he was climbing the stairwell of his apartment block. His door was locked, and it took him some time to find the key. When he let himself in, it looked as if little had changed: bed still unmade, far window open, his daughter's toys in a basket by the bathroom.

'Hetal,' he called out. 'I'm here. It's me.'

He stopped. In the middle of the bed was a sheet of paper, torn roughly from one of his notebooks. He grabbed it, held it to the light.

'Dearest one,' he read, and had to stop, the tears blurring his vision. He wiped his eyes on his sleeve, took a deep breath, and looked down at the paper again. 'We have gone,' the note continued. 'I know you wanted us to wait, but I am frightened. People are dying here. Even the doctors have gone. I know you have to stay and I don't expect you to follow us. We both love you. Let us all pray that this thing is over soon.'

Chapter Nine

ON FRIDAY 15 JUNE 1894, three days after Kitasato's arrival in Hong Kong, a small cargo freighter sailed silently into the same harbour. No crowds awaited its arrival; no soldiers ran up the jetty to grab the hawsers as they were thrown overboard; ashore, in the shadow of the customs houses, no rickshaws began jostling each other, suddenly eager for custom. It was ten in the morning and there was a rare break in the rain. The hillsides were veined with red-clay streams, every dry gulch now frothing and coursing, sweeping down through the town where choked gutters spilled into the alleys, carrying with them every kind of debris, fruit husks, excrement.

On board, a lone white man was kneeling beside three tan-leather cases. He checked the locks, tightened the straps, then stood and gestured to the crew. As he watched, the cases were lowered by hand on to the jetty. He would have felt anxious – simply getting to this point had taken many months of patient, persistent lobbying – but also, without doubt, full of thrill and expectation. He was the last to land and, as he stood there, arms around the shoulders of his two assistants – one Chinese, the other Vietnamese – the vessel that had taken him across the typhoon-whipped South China Sea pushed off into the wind to begin its perilous voyage home.

Dr Alexandre Yersin – buttoning his coat now against
a fresh squall, sensing the jetty rock queasily under him as
he led the way to shore – had made his first attempt to
reach southern China a long two years ago. It was only
with the disease now having leapfrogged to Hong Kong –
and amid rumours of infections in ports all along India's
northwest coast, and even as far afield as Buenos Aires –
that he was finally granted permission. His arrival in Hong
Kong five weeks after the start of the outbreak – satisfying
as it must have been to at last be facing the prospect of
long-awaited frontline research – would have also been a
source of sourness: so much time wasted, so many deaths
that might, given time and dedication, have been prevented.

Yersin, who'd heard and read much of Hong Kong's
pre-eminence as an international port, was poorly prepared
for the desolation that greeted him. His first report, dated
three days later, and addressed to the Governor-General
back in Hanoi, spoke breathlessly of the colony being 'completely changed': exploring deserted streets, he had to pick
his way through tableaux of Revelation-style horror: corpses
abandoned in the middle of the street, festering mounds of
dead rats at every turn. Aware of the gruesome novelty
of what he was witnessing, he took photographs, and pasted
the prints in the back of his notebook. Beneath a shot of a
narrow street – piles of rubble in the foreground, steps
climbing away between shuttered houses – he has written
in his precise, copybook hand, '*Quartier du Taipingshan. Rue
murée et evacuée à cause de nombreux cas de peste.*' Without the
caption, and with no background knowledge, the picture
would make no sense: it is of nothing, of an absence. Yet
this is precisely the point: here is a place where human
beings once lived and from which disease has now routed

them. The peeling handbills, the splintered windows, the doors hanging crooked from their hinges: this is all that remains.

As he heaved his bags off the jetty, and stood looking out across the deserted dock, Yersin must have felt his initial excitement flagging. He was prepared for an entrance into epidemic territory, but the complete absence of any kind of reception party mystified him. By now, he felt sure, the French Consul would have received the dispatch from Saigon announcing his arrival in Hong Kong: why, then, was there no one to welcome him? With the wind getting up and rain beginning to sting his face, he shouted to his helpers, and together they hauled the cases to the lee of the customs house.

Climbing uphill from the shore, at last inside a rickshaw, Yersin would have worried about the effect of the rain: all his equipment was cased, but this was rain as he'd seldom seen it, drilling cacophonous on roofs, and he imagined it forcing through the seams of the leather, working its way into all the moving parts. The moment the embassy came in sight – tricolour snapping spray in the gale – he leant out of his rickshaw and yelled back, 'The cases! Get them under cover!'

At the door stood a solitary footman. He told Yersin to wait where he was, and disappeared inside. When he finally returned, it was with instructions that only Yersin should enter: his two servants should remain with the luggage. Inside, without the cooling effect of the downpour, the claustrophobic warmth of the monsoon soon became overwhelming, and Yersin's clothes stuck to his skin. He followed the footman along pale wood floors, down corridors rendered penumbrous by the storm outside. Finally, his guide came to a halt beside a vast mahogany door. He knocked, twisted the brass knob, and pointed Yersin inside.

Yersin, used to the pattern of petition and rebuff that had marked his dealings these last two years with the Governor-General, would by now have been feeling markedly anxious. Granted, this time he had no shortage of governmental backup: Dr Albert Calmette, Colonial Secretary of State for Health, was now on Yersin's side, and so the likelihood of a bald rejection was slim indeed. Far more likely, pondered Yersin as he sat down, was an oblique coldness, an uninterest in the goals of science, an inability to see beyond the narrow exigencies of political expediency.

He cannot have been much encouraged to find that the official behind the ostentatiously lacquered slab desk was not the Consul at all, but his stand-in, the *Chancelier d'ambassade*, Bourgeois. Whatever his shortcomings in status, however, the official had at least set time aside for Yersin. 'He was expecting me,' Yersin wrote in his subsequent report for the Pasteur Institute in Paris, and there is more than a hint of discernible relief here, a sense that, from this point on, the ride would be easier. As he listed the arrangements made so far, Bourgeois appeared to confirm Yersin's optimism. Messages with news of Yersin's imminent arrival had been sent to both the colonial secretary, James Stewart Lockhart, and Hong Kong's most senior doctor, colonial surgeon Dr Philip Ayres. Yersin should see them immediately; they would arrange laboratory space, maybe even assistants.

Bourgeois's next words, however, were heavy with warning. He leant across the desk, pursing his lips.

'And how is your English, my friend?'

Yersin shook his head. 'Not good.' The sole other language he spoke was Vietnamese, and that only after years of study and enforced application. He had never visited Britain, and from elementary school English lessons could remember only the most rudimentary greetings and farewells.

'Then you will find nothing easy. The English do not speak French, and will not comprehend your failure to speak their language. I am afraid they will think you most rude and undiplomatic.'

Yersin, accustomed as he was to setbacks, would not have seen this one coming. He would, most likely, have envisaged his arrival in Hong Kong as the start of a hopeful new chapter – dangerous, certainly, but without the bureaucratic frustrations of the last two years. Now it looked as if the pattern was set to continue. And there was more.

Bourgeois coughed and waited till Yersin looked up again. 'As you know, we are not on good terms with the British. This is not new, but it will most certainly affect your work here.' He paused.

Yersin whispered, his voice a croak, 'I understand.'

'I fear your very presence here,' Bourgeois continued, 'despite the fact that it was the British government which requested help, and that it was our own Pasteur Institute that sent you, will be construed by the Hong Kong doctors as criticism.'

Yersin felt anger rise within him. 'Criticism? How so, exactly?'

Bourgeois's voice remained soothing, low. 'Because it implies that their lot are no good. Why else would you have come this far?'

As Yersin left the embassy – 'well-informed', as he would later note, 'but terribly ill-at-ease' – he reached a hand inside his jacket. He pulled out a letter, the result of a chance encounter back in Haïphong. It was a note of introduction from 'a Dr Lefèvre' to 'Father Vigano', an Italian missionary who had lived in Hong Kong for some thirty years. This introduction – downplayed in Yersin's correspondence and reports – would prove crucial.

It is not recorded where Yersin first encountered Vigano, but one can picture the two meeting in dim candlelight, in front of the altar in Vigano's makeshift church. Or maybe Vigano was harder to track down and Yersin, with poor English and even less Chinese, was reduced to wandering the back alleys throwing out his name: 'Vigano? Anyone seen Vigano? The missionary? Father Vigano?'

The two men developed an instant rapport and Vigano, no doubt sensing Yersin's state of friendlessness, cancelled all other engagements. 'He is happy,' Yersin wrote, 'to put himself immediately at my disposition, to accompany me everywhere on my official visits and to the plague hospitals.' To Yersin's relief, Vigano was also an impressive linguist, speaking fluent English and French. As for age, Vigano must have been at least in his sixties – twice Yersin's years – for, as Yersin records, he had long ago served as an 'artillery officer in the Italian army', and in 1859 had been awarded the Légion d'honneur for his part in the Franco-Italian effort to repulse the Austrians from northern Italy at the Battle of Solferino. As a result of this, Vigano had 'retained a French heart and French feelings'.

So Yersin and Vigano set off together. They forced a frenetic pace, with the Frenchman hungry, after the two-year delay, to get to work. First, they searched out Dr Philip Ayres, colonial surgeon, and a man nearer to Vigano's age than to that of Yersin: a man so tall he had to duck to get through doorways, whose extravagant wisps of moustache – unruly and wild-tendrilled in a fashion unlikely to be permitted in any hospital today – marked him out, one would guess, as a maverick, disinclined to defer mindlessly to higher authority. It had after all been he whose strident and damning report on the state of the colony's sanitation in 1872 had been so deliberately ignored and whose gloomy predictions were now, two decades on, proving daily ever more prescient.

Ayres had been looking forward to Yersin's arrival ever since his letter from Bourgeois, and he greeted his new visitors with enthusiasm. Blithely – as it would turn out – he attempted to speak on behalf of the entire medical community, assuring Yersin 'of all assistance from the civilian doctors who form the colonial health board'.

By now, Yersin must have been questioning the validity of Bourgeois's gloomy predictions, for the rest of the day produced no encounter that was anything other than encouraging. Possibly Vigano – aware of the scale of the task ahead of Yersin – was leaving the toughest for last, but for the rest of this first Friday he introduced Yersin to a score of Portuguese and English doctors who struck Yersin, to a man, as 'friendly', 'open-minded', 'interested' and 'most agreeable'.

It would have been late by the time Yersin and Vigano finished their last call and, with the streets deserted and corner noodle bars all closed – their owners either dead or in hiding or fled to China – they'd have dined in Yersin's hotel. Already, Yersin – for the last two years a jungle explorer accustomed more to hammock than laundered sheets – would have been looking for a way out, anxious to spend his nights where he'd be researching, not sequestered away in some mute-corridored hotel, far from the epidemic streets. As yet, however, Vigano would have reminded him, no such opening had arisen. Their best bet was to wait until tomorrow, when he'd scheduled meetings with the two most influential men in the colony – Governor, Sir William Robinson, and Dr James Lowson, Superintendent of the Government Civil Hospital. If Robinson could offer nothing, no doubt Lowson – grateful to have a bacteriologist of Yersin's calibre on his side – would go out of his way to make him welcome at his own hospital. Rest assured, Vigano told Yersin, by this time tomorrow you will have your rooms.

Yersin would have slept well that night. His natural optimism – badly knocked by Bourgeois's initial doom-laden prognosis – had returned. As he replayed the day's events, he'd have recalled with relief how few of Bourgeois's remarks had proved correct. Only one matter caused him concern. Towards the end of his meeting with Frederic Stedman, an English doctor, he had been taken aside. Stedman's face had become suddenly grave, as if about to offer condolences. According to Stedman, Yersin wrote, 'a Japanese mission has been here for several days, studying plague'. And they'd already had results: Shibasaburo Kitasato, the leader of the team, had discovered a bacillus after only twenty-four hours' work. Yersin, no doubt unsettled by this, kept his feelings to himself. In none of his writings does he speak of his reaction, and so one can only guess at the depth of his disappointment and thwarted ambition. In a later update for the Governor-General, however, a changed mood had overtaken him: he now viewed this bombshell piece of intelligence in a wholly different light. In conclusion, he underscored '*bacille*', adding, in heavy pencil, a prominent exclamation mark: the 'discovery' spoken of by Stedman was now, seventy-two hours on, of dubious scientific merit.

Early the next morning, Saturday 16 June, Yersin and Vigano presented themselves at Government House. This was, and remains, an impressive piece of white-stuccoed Victorian real-estate, built at the same time and with similar ambition as the Government Civil Hospital: both speak of pomp, of the stately and unquestioned colonial project, and it is unlikely that Yersin – by now in urgent need of official assistance – would have approached the baize-smooth lawns and marble-white frontage without at least a twinge of apprehension.

He need not have worried. Sir William Robinson was far from intimidating. Official portraits show an uncanny, and rather comical, likeness to the Prince of Wales, who would succeed his mother Queen Victoria as King Edward VII some seven years later. Both men were tall, heftily built and barrel-chested; but it was their large heads and identical beards which consolidated the resemblance.

Robinson, nearing retirement at fifty-eight, was almost as well travelled as his royal lookalike. A career colonial administrator, he had served as governor in a score of other British territories, including Barbados and the Bahamas. Nothing in his career, however, had prepared him for the administrative and human catastrophe that was now Hong Kong, nor – as the most senior official responsible – for the collapse in his own standing that had accompanied it. The very day of his meeting with Yersin, the *Hong Kong Telegraph* – the colony's biggest-circulation daily – reported the latest word on the streets, 'that Sir William Robinson is really a Frenchman, and has (perhaps on account of the

Franco-Chinese war of 1884–5) gone to the trouble of
purchasing the Hong Kong governorship with the special
object of introducing the plague and deliberately killing off
the whole Chinese community'.

By the time Yersin and Vigano arrived on the Governor's doorstep shortly after breakfast, Robinson would
already have been well acquainted with the contents of the
morning papers. Yet, in Yersin's brief account, there is no
suggestion that the Governor allowed the latest flurry of
malicious gossip to affect his professional cool. Robinson,
wrote Yersin in his report for the Pasteur Institute, 'receives
us with his habitual courtesy'. This was no empty display of
manners: Robinson took the trouble personally to guarantee
Yersin 'that the doors of all the plague hospitals be open to
me'.

Robinson's influence, however, extended only so far: the
doctor with ultimate responsibility for the plague hospitals
was Lowson, the irascible skew-eyed Scot, and so it was to
the Government Civil Hospital that Yersin and Vigano
hurried first. Approaching the building's sweeping colon-
naded façade – as Kitasato had done just three days earlier
– Yersin would have had no idea how significant a figure
Lowson would prove, nor to what degree he possessed the
authority to make or break the careers of the colony's
doctors and researchers. The very last thing Yersin would
have suspected was the relish with which Lowson exercised
this power.

*

YERSIN AND VIGANO were ushered into Lowson's office
together and Vigano, as before, made the introductions.

Lowson leant across the desk, proffering a cold hand that gripped Yersin's with a surprising and unsettling force. He uttered a single French word – a lackadaisical, drawled '*bonjour*', heavy with ironic emphasis – before lapsing back into English.

'I should tell you,' he said, reaching his hands behind his head, 'that I don't have much time. It's not a good moment, right now. *Comprenez?*'

Vigano turned to Yersin and translated for him.

'But,' Yersin interjected, 'I understood that Dr Lowson would be expecting me.'

'My dear fellow,' Lowson replied, a thin smile just discernible under his moustache, 'we are in the middle of the biggest epidemic this island has ever seen. I spend my days rushing from one emergency to the next. You must forgive me if I fail to read the odd missive.'

Vigano, without interrupting, answered straight back. 'Dr Yersin is from the Pasteur Institute in Paris. As I'm sure you are aware, he is one of the world's most distinguished bacteriologists. He is here on invitation to study the plague. And the Governor,' he added darkly, 'has already assured him of every possible assistance.'

Lowson glanced from Vigano to Yersin. He nodded slowly, narrowed his eyes. 'You are aware that there is already a Japanese bacteriologist in Hong Kong? You will have heard of him, I feel sure – Shibasaburo Kitasato, a professor. He truly *is* world-famous.'

'Yes,' said Yersin, 'I have heard that he is here, and I would be happy to work alongside him. We could join forces, combine our expertise.'

Lowson shook his head. 'Professor Kitasato has come with five assistants. He is settled into his work, and – as I'm sure you have heard – he has already struck gold. He has found the bacillus that causes plague.' He paused, looking hard at Yersin. 'I wired the *Lancet* only yesterday.'

Yersin sat in silence, absorbing this latest news. On the desk a carriage clock ticked loudly. He looked at his hands. Once the *Lancet* – one of the world's best-respected medical journals – published Kitasato's findings, hearsay would become fact, with Kitasato confirmed as the plague pioneer. And yet, something in him rebelled against the speed of Kitsato's announcement. Plague had remained an enigma for centuries: surely it would not reveal its secrets in forty-eight hours?

Yersin looked up at Lowson again. 'In that case,' he said, taking a deep breath, 'I offer my sincerest congratulations to the professor, but I would still most strongly request some laboratory space of my own, ideally a room in one of the plague hospitals.'

'I think,' Lowson replied, 'that Professor Kitasato has taken the last available space. As you will understand, I made sure he had the very best.'

Yersin, disappointment turning to fury, rose abruptly to his feet. Vigano reached out, put a hand on his arm. '*Attends*,' he murmured. To Lowson, gently, he said, 'A simple room would suffice. Dr Yersin, as you know, is travelling alone. He is not greedy for space.'

Lowson drummed his fingers on the table top, his long nails loud as tap shoes on the lacquer. He addressed a point over their heads, his focus jittery. 'Not this morning. Impossible. Later on I will take you around the hospitals. Afternoon it'll have to be. Three o'clock. And now,' he finished, standing up from his desk and, without pausing to shake hands, striding towards the door, 'you will have to excuse me. I have an epidemic on my hands.'

*

OF ALL THE CLUES to the strange brew of passion and misanthropy that was James Lowson, his diary for 1894 was the most compelling. The original was guarded by his granddaughter in Australia but a sole microfilm copy existed in the archives of a small medical science museum in Taipingshan – a building erected in the aftermath of plague as the colony's first and desperately needed pathology institute. Through the densely written pages – and the careful paste-ins of endless newspaper cuttings – comes a sense of a man in the grip not only of a thrilling emergency, but also of his own powerful prejudices, his own quite particular and unbending view of the world.

The difference in attitude and approach towards Kitasato and Yersin was immediately obvious, and – though Yersin's writings led one to suspect as much – shocking in its lack of professional impartiality. For 14 June, the entry read, 'Kitasato discovered bacillus. Kitasato and Aoyama to dinner – good chaps.' In the coming weeks followed the record of numerous other dinners with the Japanese team, as well as the odd 'tiffin', officer-corps slang for snack. Yersin received no such hospitality. Whenever he made an appearance in Lowson's journal it was seldom by name: on 16 June, the day the Scot grudgingly assented to show him the different plague hospitals, the entry read baldly, 'Took Frenchman around.' Within the space of a few hours, Yersin had been reduced to a faceless nonentity, distinguishable only by nationality. His presence, Lowson's cursory scribble implied, was an irritation, although thankfully one that could be quickly knocked aside. He would have to fend for himself.

The reasons for Lowson's animosity towards Yersin were harder to gauge, but there were clues. Despite a calculated and sustained tone of scientific detachment, his fifty-eight-page official report on the epidemic expended considerable energy justifying his own failure to make any kind of discovery. 'It may be thought,' he argued, 'that we surely had enough time to make some efforts in the direction of discovering bacilli. I can only say that after a day of from twelve to eighteen hours' hard and exciting work in the trying heat of a Hong Kong summer none of the men who had to bear the brunt of medical supervision, and who had to look forward to a prolonged mental strain, were much inclined to start work with the microscope by gaslight.' His labours and those of his doctors were the real work, necessitating bravery on a scale not required of the men of science. 'In the Egyptian epidemic in 1843 half of the French physicians in Cairo perished from the plague; and in the Russian epidemic in 1879 . . . the first three medical men who were in attendance on the sick died, as did numerous attendants. These were the somewhat appalling figures when the epidemic broke out.'

As he warmed to his theme, his sense of resentment became more pronounced. 'Some of us,' he complained, 'must regret that our time, being taken up by practical work in connection with the treatment of the plague – for which no fame is secured – we had so little time to look to the more purely scientific side of the question.' The key phrase – 'for which no fame is secured' – seemed the crux, and Yersin – in Lowson's eyes by far the less impressive of the two foreign scientists – made an easy target for his bitterness.

Unlike Kitasato, Yersin was profoundly dissimilar to Lowson: where the Frenchman was socially reserved, Lowson was gregarious, indiscreet, a successful and popular sportsman, who spent most evenings – at least before the outbreak of plague – drinking at his club or dining with friends. As his diary shows, he had little time for difference, for those whose approach was more circumspect than his own. An official who disagreed with Lowson on an aspect of treatment is described as 'not listening . . . I cleared out'. Later, Lowson accuses the members of the sanitary committee of doing 'nothing but complaining and making idiotic comments', while 'we doctors were fed up at having all the dangerous work to do and never one minute off duty'. Even Governor Sir William Robinson does not escape Lowson's vitriol: at one point, for reasons unspecified, he and the Colonial Secretary, James Stewart Lockhart, are described as 'making themselves obnoxious – bloody fools'.

It is quite possible that – far more than all this – Lowson was in plain language a snob, who found himself pawing the ground in front of the statesman scientist Kitasato, but who simply did not register the presence of Yersin as in any way significant. Kitasato was a welcome guest, Yersin an interloper; Kitasato merited his wholehearted support and hospitality, Yersin manifestly did not. There was no doubt in Lowson's mind who would ultimately prevail: how, he'd have asked himself, could anyone in their right mind equate this mumbling, undersized Frenchman with the brooding, mysterious genius that was Kitasato? There was simply no contest.

*

AT THREE THE SAME Saturday afternoon – five weeks into
the epidemic, with some eighty thousand Chinese now
having fled to China and the death rate showing little sign
of slowing – Yersin and Vigano presented themselves once
more at the door to Lowson's office. He, no doubt keen
to shoehorn the promised hospital tour into as short a
period as possible, ushered them immediately into waiting
rickshaws. They careered down the hairpins from the
Government Civil Hospital as the monsoon swept in again.
Out on the rain-smooth water, huddled in the back of a
part-covered rowing boat commandeered as a ferry, Yersin
saw white dolphins, oblivious to the chaos and panic in the
world above, chasing their wake.

They came alongside the *Hygeia*. Yersin's first
impressions have not survived – in his Pasteur report he
remarked only that there were eight patients on board, all
English soldiers, making it something less than a quarter
full – but it is hard to imagine that the very fact of a hospital
ship, especially one this empty, did not strike him as at least
a touch surreal. He'd have noted the long line of aching-
black, featureless windows, the lack of any open deck space,
rust bleeding from the hawsehole. Glancing up at the roof,
he'd have wondered too about ventilation: the stovepipe
chimneys were clearly for braziers; the three rooftop vents
appeared to be seized shut. He'd have looked back, across
the quarter-mile of water they'd crossed to reach the vessel,
and wondered just how much of a function such an isolated
hospital could ever perform. In the hours between his earlier
dismissal by Lowson and their three o'clock appointment,
he'd walked the deserted streets of the central district, and
what he'd seen would have convinced him that doctors

should have been in the heart of the epidemic, not sequestered away out here, in this floating mausoleum.

Hygeia had a wedge of steps, riveted in place, from deck
to water, and Yersin and Vigano stepped from the gunwale
of the rowboat and climbed towards the half-sized door in
the ship's side through which Lowson, a moment earlier,
had disappeared. Once inside, their eyes would have taken
a while to adjust to the gloom. Then he heard the intermittent groaning; the whisper of doctors and attendants;
the rubber-wheeled hum of the medicine trolley; saw the
foetal-crouched, shivering forms. Lowson, in conversation
with another doctor, let Yersin and Vigano stand ignored
at the entrance before turning abruptly on his heel and
hurrying them around the beds.

The *Hygeia* patients, Yersin wrote, 'appeared to be convalescing'. All eight, having made it through the first week
of infection, were likely to recover: a sample highly unrepre-
sentative of the *pestifières* as a whole, some eighty per cent
of whom never survived. Yersin paused beside each one,
lifting aside the bedclothes and bandages to examine the
buboes, the bruise-dark swellings in groin and neck and
armpit that were the distinguishing marks of bubonic
plague. At each slight movement, even the final lifting of
the bandage, Yersin was struck by the flash of pain in the
men's eyes, the limbs tensing then loosening, the hand grab-
bing at the sheet and bed-frame. Within five minutes, ten
at the outside, he would have finished his round; at the
door, Lowson was waiting impatiently; the boatman's hands
were already on the oars.

For half an hour, heading into the wind, they kept
parallel to the shore and made slow progress. Yersin wanted
to offer assistance to their boatman, who was continually

knocked sideways by ever-bigger waves, but Lowson made it clear that the three Europeans should be above such petty acts of charity: he'd ordered Yersin and Vigano into the covered stern, from where he now barked instructions at the boatman in nursery English, clapping his hands for emphasis. As they progressed, he shouted out the names of landmarks on the mainland.

'Government House, Harbour Office, GPO,' he hollered above the crash of waves against the bow. He gesticulated wildly. 'Peak Tram, Happy Valley, Kellett Island gunpowder depot.'

Yersin found himself drifting into reverie, this ponderous boat passage the first time for reflection since his arrival. They were heading for the northwestern tip of the island, to the Kennedy Town district, where – in the building once used as a police station, now commandeered as plague hospital – Kitasato and his team were at work. Lowson had indicated, though pointedly made no promise, that there might be a room here where Yersin could base himself, and this appealed to Yersin. As former pupils of Louis Pasteur and Robert Koch, he and Kitasato would be sure to adopt quite different approaches to research, but this could only benefit the work: they'd be targeting the same problems from different but complementary angles.

They landed with a jolt, riding heavy against the pilings of the Belchers Bay jetty. Along the entire length of the dock there was only one other vessel moored, and it took a brief glance for Yersin to know its purpose: coffins were being unloaded, passed from ship to land along a line of barefoot, shaven-headed workers, their stripped torsos polished with sweat, ragged soaking trousers held up with twine. Beyond the jetty, on a patch of rutted mud, stood a horse and cart, the animal with its head hung low, mouth afroth. A track led away from the shore, climbing up a sparsely wooded hillside. Halfway up, Yersin spotted tiny figures, working at what seemed like a chalk quarry: the excavations had exposed a pure-white scar in the landscape.

'Burial pits,' said Lowson, watching him. 'Quicklime. We get them under as soon as we can.'

From the jetty they walked, turning their heads from the stench as they passed the coffin cart, aware suddenly of a crescendo whine of insects, turning to see a crust of flies around the lid of the topmost coffin. The hospital, some fifteen minutes later, was unmistakable: a red cross flying from the flagpole; a group of nurses in white dresses and starched caps in conversation on the grass at the foot of the main steps. From what Yersin could see, a veranda encircled the entire building, and on this extra cots had been assembled. The building was of brick – a rich clay red, darkened by the rain – and two storeys. It reminded him of the country lodge of a Vietnamese colonial official.

The nursing staff, Lowson explained as they approached, were all European, and the patients billeted here were those happy to accept Western medicine; the rest – the majority, all those who had refused to go under the scalpel – being divided between the nearby glass factory and the Tung Wah hospital, based in Taipingshan, the epicentre of the epidemic.

The moment he stepped through the main entrance, Yersin knew that this was where he wanted to work. From the very first glance inside, it seemed the antithesis of the cramped and diseased central district, with its weeping, glassy-eyed corpses and gutters blocked with dead rats, with its abandoned houses and smoking pyres of clothes and broken chairs. What he was looking at now was the model of a field hospital: polished wood floors, large windows affording an ample breeze, a surfeit of beds. In a far corner, under an open window, he even saw a patient smiling at the nurse bending over him.

*

A POLICEMAN WAS standing in front of a large, dark-wood door. Lowson stopped, shook his hand and, turning, pointed at Yersin, then Vigano. The policeman nodded, sombre. Yersin could see his jaw muscles working, flickers of tension under the skin. He noticed his revolver, his riot baton, the fatigue in his eyes. The policeman nodded once more and picked a key from the loop on his belt, then slotted it into the lock. He opened the door, directing Yersin and Vigano to follow Lowson.

They were in a dark passageway now, windows shuttered. Yersin heard the key turn in the lock behind him then Lowson, at the front, splutter what sounded like curses. He heard him rattling at something, then, cursing again, give up and knock loudly.

'Kitasato!' Lowson shouted, but before he had a chance to cry out further the door opened and light flooded into the passage. Yersin could see a diminutive, bespectacled Japanese, whose hand was now being vigorously pumped by Lowson. He wore a white cotton suit, surgical mask and gloves. Behind him were workbenches with microscopes and slide trays. Just visible around the doorjamb were the feta-white feet of a corpse, tag tied around a toe.

Yersin and Vigano followed Lowson into the room. Two Japanese researchers in long white coats were bent over the corpse. The chest had been sheared open and Yersin saw the astonishing scarlet of the interior organs. One of the men was working away with a scalpel, up to his forearm in blood, while the other held out a white enamel bowl. It seemed to Yersin, though he was too far away to be sure, that they were extracting slices of lung, an approach which perplexed him: why, he puzzled, would any scientist have imagined the mechanism of the disease to be found in the lungs, rather than in the plague swellings themselves?

In his Pasteur report, Yersin made special note of his astonishment. 'I am surprised to see,' he wrote, 'that they are not even examining the bubo; rather, they are minutely investigating the heart, the lungs, the liver, the spleen, etc.' This bewilderment doubled when he saw Kitasato go on to place the samples under his microscope. Announcing that he could find no evidence of 'his bacillus, [Kitasato] declares that the patient died of typhoid fever and not the plague!'

If the duration of his first encounter with Kitasato is unknown, what is clear is that, the longer it went on, the more sceptical Yersin became of his competitor's approach. Doubtless, the intensity of his feelings of rivalry made it inevitable that he should look for flaws; certainly it would seem that, from the moment he first confronted Kitasato – deliberately belittling him in his notes as *Monsieur*, rather than *Professeur* – he was determined to strip away the aura of invincibility with which Lowson, all day, had been lovingly garlanding him. In the end, however, he could easily have afforded a less defensive posture: invited by Kitasato to have a look through the microscope, Yersin saw not only the typhoid bacilli that Kitasato had claimed were there, but smaller, scarcer bacteria. For the first time, a buoyant note, a palpable sense that the prize is yet to be seized, enters his writing. 'I refrain, however, from any comment.' There is triumph here, excitement, and not a little relief.

Encouraged to find himself suddenly on a more level footing with Kitasato – notwithstanding the latter's settled and impressive surroundings, and the industrious bustle of his assistants – Yersin, emboldened, approached him directly. Of this, the pivotal moment of their relations, a detailed first-person account is needed, but the only one that survives – that of Yersin – runs to a mere three hundred words. In all Kitasato's writings there is scant mention of Yersin, and one can only conclude that he was consciously airbrushed from the photograph of memory, as if all Kitasato noticed was himself, his own work and his own circle of intimates: even Lowson, his most loyal champion, is referred to at one point as 'a British quarantine officer', a post that he not only never held, but which was also way beneath him. In Yersin's account, there follows the telling detail that, 'as [the Japanese] know neither English nor French, I try to converse with them in German'. This was Yersin – a shy man, remember, who would concoct elaborate excuses rather than attend a cocktail party – making a deliberate effort to extend a cordial hand to Kitasato. He spoke in the spirit of scientific collaboration, knowing his German to be worse than ropy, yet confident that Kitasato would reply in the same willing and cooperative spirit.

What he would never have expected was ridicule. Barely had he finished his stumbling opening remarks than the Japanese scientists, without even the most cursory response, began 'laughing among themselves'. And then, to a man, they turned their backs on him.

Chapter Ten

HE COULD SMELL the kerosene before he reached the door; by the time he was on the street, a wad of rupees in his back pocket, leaving home with nothing but the clothes in which he stood, the reek was overpowering. The road had cleared a little since dawn, and the air was charged with a different atmosphere: less panic, more fury. Vehicles were actually moving now, albeit at a crawl: scooters carried whole families, a flatbed truck the residents of an entire apartment block. Across the street, cutting through the growl and whine of engines, came the sound of breaking glass.

Mohanlal elbowed through, ducking under the neck of a motionless, oblivious cow. He heard the splinter of glass again, followed by a yelp that sounded like war: pure vengeful emotion. His way barred, he climbed over the bonnet of a Toyota, the metal scalding his hands, sensing the bumper give underfoot as he sprang to the far pavement. Looking up, he saw that what had once been the surgery of his neighbour, Dr Ramesh Shah, was now a disintegrating shell, the windows gone, door shredded. Inside, glass was strewn across the desk and the waiting-room chairs. A man was pouring kerosene from a soda bottle, his face expressionless. He lifted the bottle, sprayed an arc across the wall.

'Stop!' Mohanlal screamed. 'What are you doing?'

Another man, axe in hand, met his eye. His lips were wet, his teeth red. 'He is a rich man, and a coward. He deserves nothing.'

Mohanlal stepped into the destroyed surgery; glass, like so much harmless candy, crunched underfoot. 'You can't burn it down. The whole block will go. Give me the kerosene.' He held out his hand. The whole scene seemed suddenly out of reach, beyond surreal: he felt nothing, not the terror he'd expected, just a sense of being underwater, every sound muffled. He watched his hand, the kerosene, his adversary, all this in silence. Then suddenly, and to his astonishment, the other man shoved the bottle at him, and the sound burst riotously back on. Everyone was shouting. Mohanlal, clutching the bottle, his shirtfront drenched, stepped backwards, almost tripping, on to the sidewalk. Before he'd had a chance even to turn, the men inside were bent to work again. Mohanlal saw the axe raised high, a flurry of papers, a chair in midair. And he ran.

His head was full of overheard conversation, fragments that turned his normally dispassionate reporter's brain to panic: 'No one is left', 'If you stay, you die', 'You know how much the bus . . .', 'Forget the train', 'But the doctors . . .' Then his attention was drawn by a crowd gathered on a patch of garbage-strewn wasteland. Those people, in dramatic contrast to everyone else, were stationary, gathered in a circle, facing inward: their very stillness was astonishing, and he found himself breaking away from the road to pick his way across the mud towards them.

Closing in, he glimpsed the flash of a spade, and his first thought was: cover-up. Someone has died, and they're interring him, they're trying to avoid being hospitalized themselves. But when he stood at the edge of the group, and looked through the heads to the centre, he saw no sheeted corpse, just a growing hole in the ground.

'We're burying it,' said one man. He coughed: his mask filled, collapsed. Mohanlal thought he saw blood on the material, and he knew what this meant, that the lungs were now infected. He took a step back.

'Burying?' he repeated. 'Burying what?'

'Squirrel,' came another voice. 'We found it dead. It died of plague. So we bury it.'

'And you,' shouted out another, 'are you a doctor? Are we all doomed now? Will no one get out of this place alive?'

Mohanlal, regretting the curiosity that had brought him thus far, backed further off. 'No,' he said. 'I'm not a doctor. But this is plague. You've heard that, right?'

'It is the city's fault,' barked out a voice, and to this there was a murmur of approval. 'All the garbage, the filth. No wonder we have plague.'

*

AS PLAGUE SPREAD in Surat, fear bred recrimination: we ourselves are to blame, said some; others raged at God; leftists blamed the rich, the diamond entrepreneurs and textile millionaires whose imported smoked-glass limousines were the first to hit the potholed streets out of town. The medical fraternity hardly set a better example: while the majority of doctors fled, a band of their colleagues chose instead denial, announcing a reward of three hundred thousand rupees to anyone able to demonstrate that the epidemic was not plague. To those who stayed on, like sixty-year-old Dr Sudha Trivedi, the cause of most grief was the universal lack of compassion, evidence of a dark hole, corrupted and grotesque, where the community should have had a beating heart.

As a medic herself, a specialist in health education, what wounded most deeply was witnessing fellow doctors choose their own safety over the lives of their patients. Some six years on, as she remembered those weeks – folding and unfolding her soft hands in the lap of her sari – her gaze drifted towards the window. From this height – six storeys, across the guano-spattered roofs of other apartment blocks – the Tapti was clearly visible, nearing a half-mile wide, approaching the ocean. On it were floating large white blocks, like miniature icebergs; only when the wind gusted them clear of the surface did they reveal themselves to be chunks of polystyrene. Now, in Trivedi's dark eyes, there was a pale stripe: the river's reflection, and it spoke of her connection to this place, where her grandparents and great-grandparents had lived, but whose people, more recently, had caused her such disappointment.

'It was a bad thing, a very unfortunate thing,' she said, and her voice trembled. 'When I heard that the doctors had disappeared from the city, I literally got pain in my heart. I do not expect anything of the uneducated people, but of the medical person I do expect integrity. Everyone loves his own life – that of course is the first thing – but medical people have to think of others, and that did not happen.'

Yet even the medics, in those first days, were at a loss. Trivedi's first reaction was to assume mistaken diagnosis. 'I thought it could never be plague. I'm sixty years old, and I'd never seen a plague case, so I rushed to the hospital to see the patients. Of course I had read about plague in books, but I admit I had no idea what it looked like.'

What she, in common with most Suratis, possessed in abundance, however, was a reservoir of family memories of the last time, close to a century before, that plague had struck. Stories told by her grandfather, great-aunt and father had become folklore: her great-aunt in particular, widowed before she had children, had assumed almost mythic status in the intervening decades. Trivedi's eyes sparked alight. 'She was the only woman to carry a dead body on her shoulders,' she said, raising her hands above her head to mimic her aunt's pioneering bravery. 'This was a time when nobody was ready to help anybody, but my auntie did not think like this: she served people without pause for herself. She worked like a man, and they had no remedies back then, no rescue teams, no government help. And she did not get the plague.' However, her mercy had gone hand-in-hand with a fierce sense of judgement. 'She believed that plague was God's anger at those who did not have good conduct of their lives.'

Trivedi, who stopped short of such brutal assessment, had wasted no time spreading the modern message: that plague was treatable and not an occasion for panic; that 'it was a post-flood calamity and we should not be afraid of it'; that, however fearful, people should not abandon their homes. 'Don't run around,' she told them, 'you will spread the disease.' And all the while, as she walked the streets handing out strips of tetracycline tablets, administering calm, a small voice nagged at the back of her brain: 'You thought plague was dead. You were wrong.' In the end, deprived of any other solace, she prayed that plague, once over, would never return. 'We were attacked by this disease because we were unaware of it, but we now know of its dangers: we have put our hand in the fire and will not do it again. That is what I pray.'

*

FOR CLOSE TO a week, the existence of plague was furiously contested. There was no question that the situation was extremely serious and the Surat authorities, witnessing the extraordinary scenes of panic on the roads out of town, vainly struggled for control. Mid-exodus, people were 'advised' not to leave, but to 'confine themselves' to their houses, and this very suggestion, with its note of emergency quarantine, no doubt propelled even the last remaining waverers into flight.

Conscious of the dangers of loose talk, the municipal commissioner warned that it was a criminal offence to spread rumours. In what was pitched as a precautionary measure, hawkers with roadside stalls were forbidden to sell fruit, vegetables and juices. Confusion ruled: within the space of twelve hours, and from impeccable sources, the existence of plague was first confirmed and then, with equal ferocity, denied. The confirmation came from the Surat authorities, who offered as back-up the assurance that 'plague is infectious but curable'; denial, however, issued from higher-up still, from the national government in Delhi. 'There is nothing serious in Surat,' gambled the minister with responsibility for Gujarat state – a hundred years on adopting the same ostrich approach as the Governor of French Indochina had done to Alexandre Yersin in the early 1890s – 'and if there is you can hang me.' Yet, even as these words were being spoken, the Prime Minister was ordering twenty-four-hour surveillance of Surat: a control room – this-is-Houston style – with phone banks and com-

puter screens, and instructions to document all evidence;
plague was the meltdown scenario, and it was looking ever
more plausible with each hour that passed.

*

AT THE New Civil Hospital, plague took the entire staff
unprepared. The store rooms were empty of filter masks –
not only a necessity for treating plague patients, but an
everyday surgical requirement, too. It took nine days for all
staff to be issued with them, and it was almost a month
before every doctor had a gown, gloves and goggles. Equally
serious, the hospital's laundry and incinerator were broken
down for the entire duration of the epidemic: the subsequent
inquiry noted 'open-air burning of hospital mattresses and
bedsheets used by suspected plague patients just behind the
hospital'. Few lifts were working; X-ray and electrocardio-
graph machines had been awaiting repair for weeks; and
patients' records were kept in such an illegible scrawl that
follow-up monitoring – for which home visits should have
been mandatory – was impossible.

Scarcely surprising then that, five days into the epidemic, with the hospital stretched way beyond its meagre
limits, sixty-eight patients – plague suspects all – fled the
compound. The language of those charged with their apprehension spoke of warfare, of something altogether darker
and more malevolent. 'They are living bombs,' muttered
the chief of the health department, 'and we have to locate
them at any cost.'

*

IN THE back alleys off Ved Road – where the first corpse,
weeping blood from nose and eyes, was stumbled upon –

the chaos of those first few days was vividly and swiftly remembered. Until that point, plague had been a disease of the past, no more relevant to the residents of Ved Road than the last Viceroy, or Gandhi: a point of drama from history, now long forgotten. Even a young doctor such as Chetan Acharya, walking today through the plague district, admitted that, the moment he heard the first rumours, he'd gone straight to his dictionaries of disease. The rest of the population, with no information but the whispers of neighbours on which to rely, chose flight; the bolder few, and those with no place to go, opted to stay, and what action they took spoke more of hope than of either knowledge or experience.

For Hitnath Zha, an orange-robed, sandalwood-scented social worker, the cause of plague was rats, and he'd spent the small hours of the first plague night setting traps all around the house. For the entire next week, in concert with his neighbours, he'd boycotted fresh fruit and vegetables. The one rat he managed to snare he bagged and carried far from his house, burying it deep in waste ground, working in the heat with mask and gloves, the earth soft and dark as molasses after the rain and the flood.

Plague hit Surat at its weakest moment. The floodwater had barely receded; corpses of drowned animals lay like abandoned meal sacks in the roads and alleys; mud lay six inches deep on the living-room floors of houses. Yet with entire neighbourhoods suddenly on the move, and every sense of safety long gone, there were still those who chose to remain. A young man and his grandfather – the same sad-dog eyes, hawk nose – recalled their own decision.

'We had nowhere to go,' the younger man said, shrugging. 'I am born and brought up in Surat, my grandfather too. The migrants, the diamond and textile workers, they could all go back home, but for us, this is our home.'

Had they been more watchful or knowledgeable, they might have spotted the warning signs: the floodwaters whose grimemark even now, six years on, was visible halfway up the concrete walls; the sewage-corrupted grain silos; the vultures that perched high in the telegraph poles. It was not until their community night-watchman was found unconscious on a neighbour's doorstep one morning – only an hour from death, his gums and lips bleeding and livid – that a far worse scenario began to present itself, a situation for which no one was in any way prepared.

The usual theories proliferated, all uncannily reminiscent of the fourteenth century: plague had broken out because drinking water was poisoned by sewage; because of some effluent secreted by rat corpses; because of an unnamed airborne contaminant. And, as in the Middle Ages, those that fled – the majority – were stoned as they entered each new town. For days, their calves bandaged against the maulings of wild dogs, they went without food. For water, they pillaged wells or, late at night, stole into backyards, emptying faucets straight into their mouths.

*

IT WAS NEARLY DARK. Dr Chetan Acharya was talking as he drove, lights off. He turned off Ved Road on to a rough track and the light seemed suddenly to fade.

'All this,' he said softly, 'it is a very recent memory for the people here. At least ten lakhs, one million people, were affected by the flood alone, even before we were hit by plague. It was a terrible calamity. And what coverage did that receive in the world media? Nothing. If just ten people in the US had been caught in floods, just imagine the cameras, the commentators.'

He fell silent. Ahead was a dry riverbed, then a steep bank. Further on was a landfill site, garbage glowing palely. The light was almost gone. He stopped the car.

'I am lost,' he said. He turned the headlights on and a cow, dazzled by the glare, stared back. On every horizon electricity glowed orange: there was no sunset. Dark shapes loomed, then receded. He shoved the car into reverse and turned. His tracks were still visible in the dirt.

Chapter Eleven

MORE THAN ANY OTHER DISEASE, plague has changed the course of history. It has surged across continents, leapt oceans, operated according to its own ferocious and apparently random rules. For thousands of years, it remained a mystery, and there is today still much about its mechanism that is unknown. Of all diseases, plague – even in this age of Aids, Ebola, resurgent tuberculosis and malaria – still retains a unique potency, and for good reason. Europe, in the fourteenth century, lost a quarter of its population to plague, and this in turn altered the continent's entire economic structure: before 1346, overpopulation had meant that only skilled professionals – teachers of Latin, farm managers – were in short supply; come plague, there were suddenly no men to drive ploughs nor sow and harvest crops. Professors became carpenters, linguists became wheelwrights. Two and a half centuries later, plague scythed down half a million in northern Spain: subsequent outbreaks in the seventeenth century doubled that total, bringing Spain's seemingly unassailable political and economic dominance to an abrupt end.

The history of plague is the story of humanity – wild and unpredictable, bloody and brooding, intimately connected to the lives of the animals that serve and stalk us and to the crops we cultivate, dependent upon season and rainfall and ecological disturbance, but not without the possibility of redemption, cure and deliverance. Plague has been part of the English lexicon ever since the publication of the King James Bible in 1611, though whether the 'plague of the Philistines' referred to in chapters five and six of the first book of Samuel was bubonic remains uncertain: what is beyond doubt is that, for seventeenth-century Europeans, with three centuries of plague behind them, no disease held greater potency, and it would, therefore, have been the inevitable translators' choice, the only credible synonym for large-scale pestilence.

In the last fifteen hundred years, references to plague have become better documented and less ambiguous. The earliest Chinese description dates from AD 610; the next, which comes some thirty years later, includes the significant observation that plague was common in Kwangtung – Canton's home province – but rare in the interior. The implication is clear: plague first hit China early in the seventh century, some two generations after it broke into the Mediterranean basin in 542. Both epidemics are now seen as part of the same continuum: the transnational outbreak known to modern historians as the first pandemic.

From the eighth century until the Middle Ages, plague remained quiescent, at least in Christian Europe, and it is this pattern of dormancy then explosion that continues to cause scientists such concern: if past behaviour is a guide to future volatility, then plague remains an uncertain, looming threat. Nowhere, it seems, is safe.

The second pandemic, which precipitated such a shakedown in European order during the Middle Ages, effected much the same in China. The numbers are astonishing: from 123 million in 1200, China's population dropped to a

mere 65 million by 1393: the intervening years had seen
a double invasion – first the Mongol hordes, then plague –
which between them had exacted a formidable destruction,
the worse, in the case of plague, for being so little understood.

Imagine a physician in Caffa in 1346, in Smyrna in the
mid-eighteenth century, in Hong Kong in 1894, in San
Francisco at the turn of the twentieth century: his town is
in the grip of plague, and he recognizes the need for action,
but has no idea what to prescribe, to advise. Only in San
Francisco – with military precision and muscle, backed
by the weight of federal government – was anything
approaching the right course taken. In all earlier outbreaks,
efforts at control had been furious but wayward: the only
common factor was the desire to do *something*, since the
alternative – despair, apathy, nihilism – was unimaginable.
By the early nineteenth century, the thinking had simplified:
plague, as an 1819 select committee in the British parliament
reported, was 'a disease communicable by contact only',
and what modifications this hypothesis underwent over the
next hundred years were at best nominal: instructions to
plague fighters in Bombay in 1898 defined the disease as
'essentially associated with unsanitary conditions in human
habitations, the chief of which are accumulations of filth,
overcrowding and absence of light and ventilation'; it was
'mainly conveyed from place to place by individuals in
their person, clothing and personal effects'. These, and
thousands of other such claims, were at least partial truths,
and quarantine, it was hoped, was a broad enough
approach to be effective. The requirements were certainly
rigorous: ships arriving from ports suspected of plague had
to anchor in a scheduled port for forty days, during which

time no communication with land was allowed. Yet plague
– through mechanisms that remained frustratingly opaque
– continued to elude such border controls.

Its longevity as a threat and its refusal to surrender up
its secrets meant that plague long ago became a routine
human crisis – no less to be feared, but at least able to be
anticipated. Writers as diverse as the fourteenth-century
poets Giovanni Boccaccio, Geoffrey Chaucer and William
Langland all treated plague, and the very real possibility of
sudden and unglorious death, as the mirror-side of life: an
act of God, like a freak storm or drought.

There were other consequences for literature: scholars
have even suggested that the decay of Latin as a *lingua
franca* among educated Europeans, and the rise of national
languages as a medium for serious writing, were hastened
by the death from plague of swathes of clerics and teachers.
Artists, too, became bleaker in their vision: the serenity of
Giotto was replaced, in the work of many painters, by the
common use of motifs such as the 'Dance of Death'. The
effervescence and buoyancy of the thirteenth-century –
which saw the joyous construction of many of Europe's
finest cathedrals – gave way to a more troubled, interior
age.

Chapter Twelve

Ridiculed by the Japanese, barely tolerated by James Lowson, Yersin found himself in a deeply uncomfortable and uncertain situation. From his brief tour around the former Kennedy Town police station – in which Kitasato's team were now so generously accommodated – he'd have quickly registered that, despite Lowson's earlier indications, no rooms remained unoccupied. He needed laboratory space, and required it in or close to Kennedy Town, since it was here, on the western corner of the island, that the plague pits were located and here, therefore, that he stood most chance of gaining access to the corpses he needed for autopsy work. Faced with a suddenly implacable Lowson, he insisted that provision be found for him. He spoke of his own medical duty, of the obligations of doctors in general, coming close as he dared to direct accusation. Then, quite unexpectedly, Lowson relented.

There was, he told Yersin, one possibility, but it would require a restricted and modest use of space. On the first-floor gallery – an area through which orderlies and other hospital staff could freely pass – there was just enough room to set up a workbench. Yersin, he said, could work there. With that – just a gesture roofward to indicate the approximate location of Yersin's quarters – Lowson swept from the cool-wood interior to the monsoon heat outside, his white coat afloat behind him, barking for his rickshaw, relieved, at least for the moment, to be rid of his troublesome Frenchman.

For the next few days, Yersin saw little of Lowson, and even less of Kitasato who, though at work in the same hospital, kept himself and his team cloistered away in their rooms, scurrying out only at dusk, back to their hotel. Doubtless Lowson, as the doctor in charge of the plague hospitals, was extremely pressed: it was his responsibility to oversee all treatment, discuss and decide on diagnoses, to steer a diplomatic course between the open distrust and venom of the Chinese and the righteous Victorian determination of the colonial authorities. It was also he – as his twenty-three-page letter at the end of May to the Foreign Secretary in London showed – who was behind such questionable practices as eucalyptus-oil-soaked handkerchiefs for all 'sisters and attendants'; whose research had led him erroneously to conclude that plague was 'not infectious or contagious', and 'probably more chemical than bacterial'; who had struggled so hard to recruit hospital attendants after 'the Chinese amahs and boys [had] simply fled'; and for whom the burden of work was so great that 'only by slaving night and day [was I] enabled to carry on'.

Yersin rose early the following morning, two days since his arrival on the island, anxious to begin work as soon as possible. The day, however, did not start well: at eight o'clock, he came out of the hotel with his pressure sterilizer and microscope cases and, as he waited on the pavement for a rickshaw, one of his assistants fled down the street. Dust eddied in his wake; a lone soldier, out on a morning patrol, shouted after him but made no effort, in the already claustrophobic heat, to follow. Yersin's first reaction was to

assume innocence – 'at first I think that [he ran away] out
of fear for the plague' – but there must have been something
in the Chinese boy's demeanour – a failure to meet his eye
that morning, shirt collar too soon sodden with sweat – that
made him reassess. Instinctively, he reached inside his jacket
for his wallet. Opening it, the boy's abrupt flight made
perfect sense: seventy-five piastres, a substantial wad of
notes, were missing.

On the way to Kennedy Town, Yersin turned over the
incident in his mind. From his writings, surprisingly little
rancour is detectable: for a prouder man, such a betrayal
might have triggered a vengeful hunt for the culprit;
Yersin, focused solely on the work ahead, saw only
'inconvenience . . . I was counting on this Chinese person
as an interpreter with his compatriots'. Yet one wonders at
his professed sangfroid. Friendless enough before, Yersin
would now – whatever his subsequent editorializing – have
felt exposed as never before. He could rely on no one, not
even those in his pay, and for any human being – no matter
how assured – there can be few bleaker realizations.

The whole of that day, Sunday 17 June, Yersin worked
virtually alone, at his side his sole remaining retainer: the
Vietnamese boy who'd accompanied him on his later jungle
expeditions. Over the next few hours, he took delivery of a
number of guinea pigs and mice – experimental animals,
all intended for the same unlovely end – and installed his
equipment. Recalling the gleaming ranks of optical and
surgical instruments that had proliferated along every inch
of Kitasato's research space, Yersin must have felt acutely
his own conspicuous lack of hardware. He had microscopes and scalpels and autoclaves – two-piece, cylindrical
pressure sterilizers, their curved steel dulled to pewter by the

humidity – but, laid out in front of him, the entire array would have occupied less than half the bench-top.

His next step was obvious, and should have been straightforward. 'More than anything,' he wrote of this moment, 'I would like to perform an autopsy.' Only by excavating the plague swellings from a fresh corpse, and sliding a smear under the microscope, could he begin investigating the infective agent. He'd have heard of the difficulties in obtaining fresh corpses – Lowson's taste for the macabre was such that he'd have had few qualms about detailing the lengths to which the Chinese were likely to go to prevent dissection of their dead relatives – but was also aware that Kitasato, as far as he could tell, had no shortage. Once set up, therefore, Yersin would have lost no time in dispatching his assistant to the doctor in charge of the temporary plague hospital. His request would have been simple: the next death you have, ensure I get first look.

And then he'd have waited, confident that, within a couple of hours at most, he'd be standing, scalpel glinting between fingertips, over a bloated and gaseous blue-black corpse. He'd have learnt of the symptoms from Lowson, who'd have listed them with characteristically lurid relish. It is clear from the reports that the Scot went on to write – one for the Foreign Secretary in London, another for the Governor – that the more extreme the case, the more acute his sense of thrill. The bubo, 'present in ninety per cent of cases, is generally exquisitely tender'; the tongue furred white, turning 'absolutely black before death'; victims were pictured lying on 'miserable sodden matting soaked with abominations', their tongues 'black and protruding', limbs in spasm. So Yersin would have been expecting the worst, the most gargoylish contortions in death, the most foetid, subhuman odours.

What he could not have expected was the response he got. Within minutes, his assistant reappeared with the news that '[no autopsies] will be carried out today'. His reaction to this rebuff is not recorded. Even at this stage, it is possible that – despite Lowson's undisguised favouritism – Yersin's suspicions were not yet aroused, and indeed he was, before long, given an encouraging update. A doctor approached carrying a tray of test tubes containing blood samples from patients: he could at least start somewhere.

For the rest of that first day, Yersin blurred slides with blood and squinted at them through his microscope, inching the deepening purple smears under the bulb of his lens till his eyes had trouble focusing and he became too hungry to continue. Sometime – maybe this day, possibly later – he broke from his work and walked outside, following the death carts to the plague pits on the lower slopes of Mount Davis. He had his box camera with him and here, as elsewhere, and as if aware of the momentousness of the times, he recorded what he saw. The print that survives of the burial ground seems artificially dark, like those early-movie attempts at creating the effect of night, but shows clearly the industrial scale of the burial programme. A pile of new-quarried and chalk-white slabs occupies the immediate foreground. The incline rises sharply and, cut into the receding hillside, there are row upon row of gravestones, divided level from level by broad steps of freshly turned earth. To the uneducated eye, the gradations look as neat as rice paddies in the dry season, awaiting rain and hoe.

Returning to his laboratory, Yersin bent over his microscope once more. By now, he had examined the blood from 'several patients'. The results had been uniform and negative. Nowhere did he discover anything out of the ordinary – no bacillus, no microbe, no infective agent.

Kitasato, by contrast, was at that very moment claiming spectacular results. In his report of 15 July, addressed to the Japanese Interior Minister and later published in the *Tokyo Medical School Journal*, he records 14 June – when Yersin's boat was still a full day's sail from Hong Kong waters – as the date of his first autopsy. The dissection was carried out by his pathologist, Professor Tanemichi Aoyama, on a corpse some eleven hours old. Lungs, spleen, liver, buboes and blood from the heart were removed. In all, Kitasato wrote, 'I found a great deal of bacilli'. He filled a syringe with the blood and injected it into two laboratory mice: they died two days later. 'Day after day,' Kitasato recorded, 'I took blood from plague patients for examination and found the same bacilli.'

Kitasato was triumphant: the mechanism of plague, the causal bacillus, was his, and already, as the ultimate stamp of official acceptance, the internationally renowned weekly medical journal the *Lancet* had accepted his findings, which were now due for imminent publication. And yet Yersin, working in parallel, examining blood samples from no doubt the same plague victims, had found no such bacillus: his own notebooks state, simply, 'no results'. Clearly they could not both be right.

Chapter Thirteen

TAKE A GENEROUS sheet of paper, coloured pens, enough space to lay it all flat. Sketch the outline of the continents, the globe unfolded. Then, with the first pen – red, for the start of the conflagration – draw a line from southern China to Hong Kong. It is 1894, and slowly, as the summer lengthens, the thin red line inches on: Amoy, Macao, Foochoo. By 1896, it has reached Bombay, and here, to signify a shift of gear, the colour changes. In purple now, lines claw outwards, to St Petersburg, Yokohama, Nagasaki. Within India, an interior web of infection grows, drawn black because the toll here is worse than anywhere, and accelerating – 55,000 deaths in 1897, 117,000 the next year, 135,000 in the twelve months after that. Before the old century has passed, a spray of yellow, like bullet tracks, hits Europe – Oporto, Lisbon, Trieste. Now we have a tangled tapestry, with the Atlantic suddenly enmeshed – Ascunción, Corrientes. A line reaches Formosa. The map is a riot of colour. Connections, like a rampantly expanding railroad network, are proliferating and fusing, spawning, always moving.

Such was the speed of the spread of the third pandemic that, within six years, every continent on earth was affected. In 1900, it struck Africa, Australia, New Zealand, London, Cardiff, Astrakhan in Russia and, finally, the west coast of

the USA. It is this last which, to this day, retains the scent
of scandal: a pattern, begun in Hong Kong in 1894, was
repeated six years on as if pre-programmed, on the far side
of the world.

*

PORT AUTHORITIES across the United States had been on
the lookout for plague ever since news had reached them
from Hong Kong. Quarantine officers were trained up and
expectant and so, when the SS *Nippon Maru* sailed through
Golden Gate on Tuesday, 27 June 1899 – at the end of
a journey begun in Hong Kong – she was immediately
impounded. The vessel was searched, and eleven Japanese
stowaways were discovered. The next day, when the crew
was shifted to Angel Island quarantine station, two of the
stowaways were found to be missing. Some days later,
their corpses, buoyed up by *Nippon Maru* life preservers,
were spotted drifting in San Francisco Bay. Autopsy results
were unequivocal: both men carried plague.

For a time, all was quiet and, week by week, public
health officials breathed easier. Then, on Tuesday 6 March,
1900 – some nine months after the two stowaways were
roped, blue-lipped and swollen, from the chop of the bay –
a man's body was stretchered, blanket over his head, from
the basement of Chinatown's Globe Hotel. Because the
victim had died alone, his death unwitnessed, an autopsy
was ordered. The physician on duty noted dark bruiselike
groin swellings and reported his suspicions to the city health
officer. Hours later, a second examination was carried out,
this time by the Health Board's bacteriologist. His report
was clear, if reluctant: the man had, in his opinion, died of
plague.

Plague had never before hit the US, and the American establishment, like the European classes in Hong Kong six years earlier, reacted with instant fury. Rather than welcome the efforts of the city to curb infection, the forces of big business instead opted for ridicule. The investigations of Federal Quarantine Officer Dr J. J. Kinyoun were lampooned in the San Francisco *Bulletin*:

> Have you heard of the deadly bacillus,
> Scourge of a populous land,
> Bacillus that threatens to kill us,
> When found in a Chinaman's gland?

Kinyoun's experimental animals were, the anonymous poet went on, 'living and thriving', which was in fact naked falsehood – two guinea pigs and a rat, all injected with plague tissue, had already died – but the pressure worked: within forty-eight hours, the hastily imposed quarantine of Chinatown was lifted.

What took its place – a sly racism, couched in the finest scientific language – was also uncannily reminiscent of Hong Kong in 1894. Soldiers were posted at strategic exit points from the city, with orders to examine anyone – but most particularly anyone Chinese – attempting to leave. By May, with the existence of plague finally accepted by the city Health Board, anti-plague regulations were hurriedly drawn up. At the very best, these were unconstitutional: one forbade 'Orientals or members of other races particularly susceptible to the disease' from using trains, streetcars or ferries. Then, as if all this were not indignity enough, the Health Board drew up proposals to evacuate all Chinese to detention camps on Angel Island and – as in Hong Kong – demolish their homes and restaurants, hotels and stores, swinging the heavy ball until nothing was left standing.

Everywhere was confusion, misinformation, obfuscation. The State Governor – at a time when the death toll was nearing a hundred – claimed that 'plague did not nor ever did exist in California' and, in January 1901, even went so far as to question Kinyoun's working methods, claiming that he had isolated the bacillus not from plague victims, but from unnamed imported cultures. Unable to leave it at that, the Governor went on to propose that the transportation of plague cultures without high-level permission should be a crime punishable by life imprisonment and that, moreover, it should be a felony to broadcast the presence of plague.

With the San Francisco Medical Society, the US Marine Hospital Service and the city Health Board all admitting the existence of plague – and the Chinese, the Merchants' Association and most newspapers issuing equally vociferous denials – rumours flew wild and unchecked. Plague, some said, had died out in the Middle Ages. According to others, it belonged to the days of Charlemagne, before the 'common people' had soap; it was, alternatively, an 'oriental' disease, peculiar to 'rice eaters'; and, concurred the majority, whatever its mechanism or cause, it certainly never attacked Caucasians.

The last victim of the first San Francisco epidemic was a 33-year-old woman from Concord, California. It was 29 February 1904, and one hundred and twenty-two people had died, in every case the cause of death the subject of strenuous dispute. The denial of plague had persisted throughout, and went to the very top: Eugene Schmitz, Mayor from 1901, even refused to approve the printing of

Health Department statistics, and did his utmost to shift from office the four members of his Health Board who continued to claim that plague was alive in the city. Then, for a while at least, plague, like a wily heavyweight, pulled back. Those who'd argued against its existence began tentatively to congratulate themselves, proving clearly that no lessons had been learned, for the disease had retreated as if of its own accord, and not as the result of any coherent hygiene drive nor any kind of concerted attempt at rat destruction. These were mistakes that America would not make again: plague, as it would yet discover, never willingly renounces a claim on new territory: once it has its claws in, it does not loosen its hold.

*

ON 18 JUNE 1894, three days after his arrival in Hong Kong, Alexandre Yersin wrote what would be the first of three bulletins to the French Governor-General in Indochina. The original draft survives and – with its hurried excisions and additions, its stutters of ink and wayward punctuation – speaks most strikingly of urgency, of an electric freshness, of the thrill of being so close to the solution to medicine's most intractable problem. It speaks, too, of the force of Yersin's ambition: two sentences outlining the work of Shibasaburo Kitasato and his team have been forcefully scored through, almost as if Yersin was trying to will his competitors into non-existence. The edited bulletin, therefore, would have reached the Governor-General with no mention of the Japanese bacteriologist.

The bulletin is also rich in description; like the imaginative novelist, Yersin knew the value of the telling detail. He writes of the contents of Chinese houses being carted to the shore and burned; of the dwellings' barbaric cleansing which saw soldiers using 'steam pumps' to 'flood them with torrents of salted water'; of the ninety-five centimetres of concrete poured over each interred corpse; of streets deserted save for the occasional shuffle-past of stretcher-bearers. 'Walking the streets of the infected areas,' he wrote, 'I notice many dead rats lying on the ground.'

*

SHORTLY AFTER DAWN that day, Alexandre Yersin had swabbed down his workbench and set up his equipment in preparation for what he hoped would be a day far more productive and revelatory than the last. As the morning passed, however, it became apparent that this was not to be: each time he tracked down the doctor in charge and requested an autopsy – his English for this phrase at least now polished and swift, no longer a target for ridicule – he was told that 'they are reserved for the Japanese'. This left him bewildered and embittered. 'I thought I had the same rights as them, but it seems I was wrong.' As yet, he assumed nothing more sinister than favouritism.

So that second day was spent much as the first: in endless microscopic examination of blood samples, each of which revealed the same uniform blank. His sense of frustration cannot have been eased by the acceleration in the rate of infection, and from the windows of the Kennedy Town hospital he'd have seen the first definite evidence of this build-up: the hasty construction of a series of grass-and-pole longhouses, which were filling with patients as fast as they could be assembled.

At some moment during the day he stood up from his microscope and walked across the patch of grass and mud that separated the two hospitals. Arriving at the new hospital, with its pallid attendants and strange and unexpected aroma of grass clippings, he would have been polite, yet insistent, and no doubt done his best to omit mention of the rebuffs he'd so far received, but here too, as if by conspiracy, no autopsies were allowed him. As before, he was permitted to take blood samples and this he'd have done wearily, returning across the uneven ground in the gathering dusk to prepare the slides with a leaden hand, by now expecting and finding nothing – no foreign agent, no squirming microscopic evidence of the parasite he knew to be there, but which he'd so far been prevented from tracking down.

The next day, 19 June, Yersin was at his workbench at five in the morning. In his notes and letters he offers no explanation for such an early start, but it is likely that he slept poorly back at his hotel, unable to find rest as he picked over the indignities of the day before. Yersin was a proud man, scrupulous in his dealings with others, and the hostility he'd encountered would have wounded and infuriated him. So the small hours found him groping for his clothes, holding a match to his bedside lantern, standing outside in the absolute dark and silence of the night while his hotelier disappeared for a rickshaw. He arrived at the hospital with dawn still an hour away, found the doctor on duty and requested – for the twentieth time – clearance for the mortuary. Once again, he was refused.

It was another five hours before the Japanese team arrived at the hospital, a fact which deepened Yersin's already pronounced sense of grievance. 'There is obviously,' he would write in his report for the Pasteur Institute, 'preferential treatment in this.' As the day progressed, his indignation found another focus, this time the stream of

casual visitors he was forced to welcome: returning from a
tour of the hospital, or from a discussion with one of the
doctors, he'd find 'people touching my laboratory animals
and my culture tubes'. For a man happiest working alone,
this was an intolerable level of intrusion, and he determined
to find a space that would offer him more privacy, more
'independence'.

*

As YERSIN WAS chewing over his next move, the Hong
Kong Governor – facing an emergency for which his
previous Caribbean postings had left him woefully under-
prepared – sat down to compose a comprehensive bulletin
to his overlords in London. From the first case of plague in
the colony, the imperial government's anxiety had been
palpable, and on 16 June, Robinson found himself opening,
no doubt with considerable trepidation, a telegram from
the Marquess of Ripon, British Colonial Secretary,
demanding news of the 'progress of bubonic plague', 'names
of any Europeans dying or attacked', a summary of 'the
effect on Finances' and confirmation that the disease had
– as was rumoured – spread from China. 'If so,' Ripon ended
darkly, 'what measures did you take against its introduction?'

Robinson, having already fired off some thirteen updates
– brief dispatches all, most often simply a tally of numbers,
totals dead or fled, names of streets and neighbourhoods
now abandoned – clearly decided that a far more expansive
account was now required. In thirty-seven numbered and
finely detailed paragraphs, he chronicled the damage so far,
and the action taken.

Lest the Colonial Secretary assume any kind of sloth or
incompetence on his part, Robinson began by stressing

the fleetness and dynamism of the legislation and medical response he'd already set in train – feats all the more impressive when one considered, ran the implication, that he'd first heard of the outbreak only on 15 May, on his return from an eight-week leave of absence in Japan. At this point, Robinson lost no time in explaining how he'd promptly set up a new sanitary committee, who 'have since acted with extraordinary energy and efficiency': hospitals had been 'at once established'.

His upbeat tone evaporated, however, when detailing the effect plague had had upon the island colony itself. 'Without exaggeration I may assert that so far as trade and commerce are concerned the plague has assumed the importance of an unexampled calamity.' The price of foodstuffs was up fifty per cent; steamers bound for San Francisco, Honolulu and Vancouver had banned Chinese passengers from boarding; mailships from England, France and Germany were not even entering the harbour, let alone taking on cargo. At least a tenth of the building stock, Robinson estimated, was destined for demolition.

Yet there was hope. From Japan – noble empire, loyal ally, whose hospitality Robinson had so recently and sumptuously enjoyed – had just arrived a party of 'experts'. The reference is brief – three lines at most – and avoids any reference to Yersin, but the implication is unmistakable. 'The Japanese experts,' Robinson wrote, 'claim to have discovered the Bacillus of the plague and the medical staff admit the claim.' Here was diagnosis, officially verified, sanctioned and approved at the highest level: the end of disease, even cure – ran Robinson's soothing subtext – was in sight.

*

ALONE AND FRIENDLESS, Yersin must have been overjoyed
at the arrival in his laboratory that day of his sole ally,
the elderly Italian missionary Father Vigano. The visit was
unannounced, and even before Vigano had had time to
pull up a chair, Yersin began unburdening himself. His
position was untenable, he said: a scientist needed quiet,
to be spared interruption, but more than this, he needed
unfettered access to research materials. And I, Yersin
lamented, have neither.

Between them, they devised a solution. 'We decide,'
Yersin wrote, 'that what is best for me is to have a little
straw hut built next to the big straw hut hospital', an
emergency shelter which had just been erected near the
Kennedy Town police station. They shook hands. Vigano
rested an arm across Yersin's shoulder; together they gazed
out in silence at the blur of white coats outside the makeshift
hospital, the grooved and beaten earth which served as
entrance area, the ever-growing pile of pale-wood coffins
outside the main door. What about permission? Yersin
queried, his initial euphoria subsiding. What likelihood was
there that the authorities, which had defied him thus far,
would suddenly grant him this kind of extraordinary planning permission? What chance at all?

It had grown late. Outside the hospital Vigano's rickshaw was waiting, driver slumped snoring across the seat.
As they stepped outside it started to rain. There was a
tremor of thunder, and the driver spluttered awake. Before
Yersin and Vigano could reach the rickshaw, water was
coursing afresh underfoot; veins of lightning flashed across
the wet ground.

*

YERSIN DOES NOT record how he was able to build his hut, but securing permission cannot have been straightforward. Red tape was a speciality of colonial government, and the stranger the request, the more desks it would have had to pass over.

His mood cannot have been much improved the next morning, Wednesday 20 June, when he learned of the contents of the *China Mail*. Under the headline 'Discovery of the Plague Bacillus', there appeared an obsequious interview with Kitasato and Aoyama. The unnamed interviewer's predispositions were plain from the start. 'It was a wise measure of the Japanese government to send these scientists here,' the article began, before proceeding at length to list Kitasato's professional credentials: his doctorate from Tokyo University, the seven years spent at Robert Koch's bacteriology institute in Berlin, the triumphant return home in 1892 and establishment of his own laboratory.

Yersin, unable to read much English, would have had to rely on Vigano for translation, and would have listened quaveringly, alert for every nuance. How much did Kitasato know? How close was he? Through the detail came hope. 'The two experts,' he'd have heard, 'have identified the Hong Kong plague with bubonic typhus,' and in that euphemism were born a hundred possibilities: that Kitasato's diagnosis was almost wholly wayward; that the Japanese team considered it likely that contagion was inhaled; that, in short, they were being congratulated on a discovery that was no such thing. Again, there was the reference to abundant plague bacilli being discovered in the blood of patients, a finding directly contradicted by Yersin's microscope work, which had uncovered no such bacteria. Kitasato and Aoyama, the writer concluded, were working on an account of their findings, publication of which was breathlessly awaited. 'Their final official report, whenever it may be ready, will no doubt prove of great value not only to the Japanese but also to the Hong Kong government; and the University of Berlin may be congratulated on having furnished Hong Kong, and we may say the scientific world, with such able, painstaking, and scientifically cautious observers as Professor Kitasato and Professor Aoyama.'

*

YERSIN, FIVE DAYS IN, began to plot rebellion. With retreat unthinkable, he and Vigano would have sat down and busked ideas, casting for a way through, some method of evading the restrictions under which Yersin's work was beginning to suffocate.

Yersin was in no doubt what he needed: unfettered access to cadavers. Yet, without official permission, there seemed no way of achieving this. All corpses were guarded by soldiers; between death and burial there was not one moment when an unauthorized person was able to breach security. Worse, the hospital mortuary was, in Yersin's words, 'a sort of cellar', outside which, for twenty-four hours a day, naval conscripts stood sentry. The plan that Yersin and Vigano eventually devised was exquisite in its simplicity, though it carried the ultimate risk: if they were discovered, Yersin would most likely be expelled from Hong Kong. His future with the Pasteur Institute would have been in shreds, his career as good as over.

Chapter Fourteen

BORDER GUARDS, customs officials, soldiers, policemen: given the right inducement, all have been known to bend the rules. Over a number days, Yersin took to passing by the naval sentries who guarded the mortuary, nodding acknowledgement after the first few times, calling out a greeting after that. Fighting to overcome his reluctance at exposing his poor English, he'd have stopped and attempted small talk, seldom getting beyond the first stock pleasantries, but sensing the sentries beginning to soften.

Returning with Father Vigano to his workbench – only to find the English wife of one of the doctors reaching and cooing into the guinea pig cage, ordering her to leave in language affronted and bellicose – he tore off a clean sheet of squared paper and began to list his expenses. The first-day theft of seventy-five piastres had left him tight for money, and the cost of building his own laboratory hut was going to restrict him further, but he now knew that he had no choice: he could wait no longer to start his autopsy work. With the authorities refusing him access, only one option remained. He would bribe the sailors guarding the mortuary. He'd take his scalpel to what bodies he could reach, then retreat fast. It was far from ideal, but he could see no other way.

Choosing to operate outside the law was certain to be

perilous. If word got out among the Chinese that Yersin was smuggling himself into the mortuary and desecrating the bodies of their relatives, he'd be lucky to escape Hong Kong alive. By the third week in June, Chinese fears had reached a histrionic pitch, and little provocation was required to ignite a fresh riot. According to the Chinese Viceroy of Canton – in a letter to the Hong Kong authorities dated just two days earlier – treatment of plague victims was barbarous: they were taken to 'the glass room, fumigated with sulphur, and given iced water to drink'. No visits from relatives were permitted. After death, victims were 'collected in a house', until they were 'buried in lime'. Anyone sick was ejected from their home, and the building and all contents 'destroyed'. The immediate efforts of the Hong Kong colonial surgeon Philip Ayres and police chief Francis May to correct these rumours – by explaining that quicklime 'only hastens the decomposition of the flesh and does not affect the bones of the dead'; that immediate burial was 'a precaution used in all civilized countries' when dealing with deaths from 'infectious disease'; that shutting up plague houses had saved 'many lives'; and that, finally, 'the people were unspeakably grateful for the forethought of the officials in thus providing for their safety' – had scant effect. Yersin would have known that by even contemplating tampering with the bodies of the dead he would be risking his life.

He approached the mortuary cautiously. The sentries, accustomed to him by now, greeted him warmly. They knew about his problems gaining access to corpses, and quizzed him on progress. Yersin and Vigano accepted these initial pleasantries, shook hands, and lowered their voices. Vigano, without prompting from Yersin, explained the situation.

How would it be, he suggested, if we offered a little money to help you with your job? Yersin, leaning close, added a further inducement: a 'tip' for each bubo that he was able to remove.

To Yersin's surprise, the sentries agreed 'immediately'. There is no mention in Yersin's notes of any bargaining having taken place, and so one must assume that the men were now on friendly enough terms with Yersin to think little of helping him out. They unlocked the mortuary and showed him in. He pulled the heavy door shut behind him and Vigano, alert for any suspicious movement, waited outside with the sentries.

Inside, in soupy darkness, Yersin groped towards the stack of coffins. Closest, he'd been told, were coffins not yet hammered shut: he had to remove the lid of one of these, conduct whatever hurried autopsy he had the stomach for, shove the lid back and run for daylight again. His eyes adjusted: head-height grilles, half-gummed with mud, threw rods of ashen light across the cellar. He rattled the first coffin: no movement. The top of the second, however, was loose and slid easily sideways. In the ghostly light, and under a rough scatter of calcium oxide, or quicklime, the face of the cadaver appeared bleached of colour. Open eyes were filled with powder pale as talcum; the cheeks were hollow; the mouth yawned open, revealing contracted gums. Against this the tongue – hardened, stuck to the roof of the mouth – was weirdly black. With no knowledge of the disease, a susceptible mind might have guessed at witchcraft, that the person who'd inhabited the body had offended the ancestors, the spirits, and so incurred the ultimate curse.

Yersin drew his scalpel, cleared the neck of quicklime. The glands here were engorged and purplish-black, and he sliced effortlessly into the cheese-soft skin, carving a ring around the swelling. The smell, even through the handkerchief he held to his face, made him cry out in shock and clutch his throat. Unsteady now, he managed to cut the bubo free and drop it into his sample tin. Holding his breath, he turned for the stairs. Back at his workbench, his heart banging in his throat, he allowed himself to look tentatively around. No one was pointing his way; nothing seemed out of the ordinary. A yelp of relief escaped from him; he lowered his head, suddenly self-conscious.

He knew that he had been lucky, but would never know quite how fine he'd cut it: that same day, most likely at the very moment Yersin was in the mortuary, James Lowson – as was his habit – paid an extended visit to Kitasato and his team. Lowson's diary, brief as ever, notes, 'Japs hard at work'. To the garrulous Scot, this would have meant a good hour or more complimenting Kitasato on his progress so far, quizzing him for an update, discussing the telegram he'd wired to the *Lancet* five days before, musing over when they might expect to see final printed proof of Kitasato's pioneer status. Lowson would also have used the opportunity once more to extend an offer of hospitality, this time a weekend dinner at the Peak Hotel, with its panoramic view over Victoria, the docks, the islands and faraway ocean.

Yersin too was now working intently, with renewed vigour and purpose. He had returned to his workbench and started simply: onto a fresh slide he smeared pus from the stolen plague swelling, and shuffled the slide on to his microscope tray. 'At first glance,' he noted '*une véritable purée de microbes*', a result which differed strikingly from the blank readings he'd obtained from the blood samples.

In the space of six hours, Yersin's mood had been transformed. After a despondent morning he was now squinting down his microscope at what had every appearance of being the elusive bacillus. His writing becomes staccato; extraneous detail falls away. Without lifting his head from the eyepiece, he made notes on the pad at his elbow. 'Squat little rods, rounded ends, some discoloration.' From the same sample he took further smears, preparing cultures with which he injected mice and guinea pigs. Then, fearing nothing, he ran back to the mortuary. Once again the sentries let him through and asked no questions. He excavated two more buboes, then returned to his workbench. By now, staring down the tube at the busy clusters – like tiny boats, seen from the height of clouds, jostling at the start of a race – he felt confidence growing. 'There is every chance that my microbe is that of the plague, but I do not yet have the right to affirm that.' The circumspection, one senses, was a professional reflex, and not true to his feelings: far more telling is that possessive pronoun, the prominent 'my'. The discovery, Yersin knew, could be his, and he wired the *Lancet* immediately with news of his findings. The only obstacle was that Kitasato was just a hair's breadth from official recognition, awaiting only the publication of the next issue of the same journal for his achievement to be endorsed. Yersin would have known this, yet there is no trace of resentment in his writing. The truth, he must have felt confident, would come out. For now, all he had to do was keep his research pure and his methods transparent. Right would prevail.

*

FROM THE STANDARDS and viewpoint of today, there is something quaint, even otherworldly, about Yersin. In the

face of enormous pressure – wrestling bandits in the Vietnamese jungle, standing alone and virtually friendless against
the Hong Kong medical establishment – he retained a
preternatural calm, in his frustration never resorting to
name-calling. He was fuelled above all, one senses, by the
conviction of the rightness of his own calling, against which
obstructions of the kind he met in Hong Kong faded into
insignificance. When he signed off letters to his mother
as 'Dr Yersin', it was an indication of the degree to which
he felt defined by his profession, his calling. Thus, in the
caption for the photograph he'd have taken of him outside
the *paillotte*, the high-roofed grass hut he was now planning,
he would write, '*Le docteur Yersin à l'entrée de sa paillotte*' –
this in the back pages of his own notebook, never a published work, and intended for but a handful of readers,
mostly colleagues who'd have needed no such information
anyway.

It took Yersin barely twenty-four hours to have the hut
assembled. Permission came through on Thursday 21 June
– and Yersin 'speedily made an agreement with a Chinese
entrepreneur' to act as builder. For seventy-five piastres
– the exact sum of which he had been robbed that first
morning – he ordered a construction big enough to serve
both as living quarters and laboratory space. The frame
would be bamboo and timber; the roof and walls grass; the
floor would sit on stilts, a good foot clear of the ground.
From the front door, sheltered from the sun by a corner-
veranda, he could look out at the Kennedy Town hospital
in which Kitasato was so comfortably installed. In the
photograph, Yersin stands white-suited, hand on hip, pro-
prietorial: despite the swiftness of its construction, the hut
has an air of permanence about it. The walls are supported

from all sides by hefty timbers, set at acute angles like guy-ropes. For Yersin, most importantly, it spelled freedom, autonomy: here he could work at his own pace, subservient to no one.

By Friday he was in, his trunk of clothes transferred by rickshaw from the hotel, his microscopes and pressure sterilizers arranged along a workbench that still smelled strongly of fresh-cut timber. Along another wall were his caged laboratory animals – mice, guinea pigs, rabbits, rats – scratching, snuffling, musky. He made a simple bed for himself – bamboo slats, a single blanket – and swept the floor. Outside, the rain appeared to be dissolving the little remaining grass, creating one long sweep of marsh. Mosquitoes, he knew, were inevitable in such 'swampy' conditions, and that first night he was 'literally devoured by them'. Yet he remained buoyant. 'This nonetheless does not stop me rejoicing that I am at last at home.'

After the initial euphoria of his first clandestine autopsy, it became clear to him that to continue his work properly he would need legitimate and full access to corpses: hurried autopsies would create rushed results, and this research was too important to be conducted illegally, in secret, and under constant threat of exposure. While the hut was still in mid-construction Yersin had applied for another autopsy, and was refused again, 'even though there were three to be done'. Aware there was a side to this that he no doubt only partially understood, but conscious too that such preferential treatment ran quite against the spirit of scientific collaboration, he took a rickshaw to the residence of the French Consul and to him, in language deliberate and measured, dictated a demand that he wished the Consul to pass onto Governor Sir William Robinson.

Two days later, after more than a week of rebuff, clearance finally came through, and the swiftness of this
turnaround raised in Yersin the same suspicions as it would
have to any alert mind. To the Governor, clearly, there was
no reason whatever why Yersin should not have been
allowed the same access to autopsies as the Japanese team,
and he lost no time in agreeing to Yersin's request. Resistance to Yersin, then, must have come from lower down
the chain of command, and the obvious figure was James
Lowson. The decision to obstruct Yersin had been taken by
him, and him alone.

Lowson's slipperiness did not stop there. On Saturday
23 June, the day Yersin received the authorization he should
have had at the start – enabling him 'to perform one out
of every two autopsies' – a yet bleaker realization dawned.
The reason that Yersin had thus far been barred from
performing autopsies was, he writes, that 'the Japanese
bought them all', though from whom he does not say. He
nowhere explains how he came to this conclusion – whether
through sentries' intelligence, a deduction made by Vigano,
or some doctor's indiscretion – but it must have hit him
hard, since it spoke more clearly than ever of Lowson's
favouritism. His disrespect for Kitasato by this point was
such that even bribery did not surprise him. 'What I am
less able to understand is that Dr Lowson could have
approved such a disloyal procedure.'

There was more. Once Yersin had started his autopsies
– building a body of evidence, methodically examining
different tissue for the prevalence of the bacillus – he
received an unexpected visit from Lowson. For the first
time, the Scottish doctor was friendly, even ingratiating.
He stooped a little as he entered the cool dark interior of

Yersin's workhut, smiling as he looked around, complimenting Yersin on the professionalism of his facilities. Then
he noticed the microscopes.

'May I?' he asked, fixing Yersin with his one good eye.

Yersin nodded, directing Lowson to a chair.

'And in this one?' Lowson queried, adjusting the eyepiece, one hand on the slide.

'The microbe,' Yersin told him, warming to Lowson's
interest. 'From the bubo.'

Lowson got up, moved to the next microscope. 'And
this?'

'The same.'

'So this is where you find the bacillus? In the bubo?
Nowhere else?'

Yersin nodded. 'And Professor Kitasato?' he began to
say, but Lowson was already at the door, composing his
goodbyes.

*

MUCH LATER, adding the footnotes to his report for the
Pasteur Institute, Yersin would look back on the unacharac-
teristic and unexpected interest that Lowson had suddenly
shown in his work. With hindsight, there was an unrelenting
logic to it – Lowson's initial opposition, the endless assistance and hospitality offered to Kitasato, then the sudden
and perplexing interest in his own research.

'Dr Lowson,' Yersin wrote, 'has shown himself too much
an ally of the Japanese. He should have been more reserved.
It is he who, after having seen my preparations, advised the
Japanese to research the microbe in the bubo. He himself
assured me, as well as several other people, that the microbe

isolated first by the Japanese did not resemble mine in any way. It was a much longer bacillus.'

He should have been more reserved.

*

THOUGH THERE WAS much that separated Yersin from the Japanese team – both in temperament and approach – in one aspect at least there was little to differentiate between them. They carried out their work with a singleminded disregard for their own safety, with a bravery that bordered on foolhardiness. In part, this was explained by their very ignorance: if plague was a disease of 'filth', then scientists operating in sterile conditions were certain to remain unaffected. Yet already this theory was looking unstable: two English soldiers, men regarded as the washed-white and upright antithesis of the pestilential 'Oriental', had died of plague – and it would not be long before two of Kitasato's team would also be struck down.

The account that survives is that of Professor Aoyama, Kitasato's pathologist and second-in-command, a man as perplexed by Hong Kong's climate – 'It is warm and there is never snow' – as he was repelled by the living conditions of the majority of its inhabitants. In some houses, he wrote, there was 'dust and filth several inches thick on the floor, matted together like felt'. Hygiene was equally lamentable: 'I have seen many women who have candidly confessed that they have not even wiped themselves down with a damp cloth for years and I saw no reason to doubt their words.' On 28 June, he sat down to lunch after a morning of autopsies 'and strangely enough it did not taste good to me'. Plague – disease of the primitive other – had laid its chill finger on him.

Aoyama lost no time in examining himself: 'pain in the left axillary space', 'several glands enlarged', 'sensation of burning heat along the whole back'. By evening, he was running a temperature of over thirty-nine degrees. For the next two weeks, he was 'practically unconscious'.

The most telling observation came near the end of the report, although neither he nor Lowson were sufficiently equipped to draw any conclusions. In many patients, Aoyama recorded, 'I often saw on the places uncovered by clothing – face, hands, the instep of the foot – round, light, red, numerous, often times somewhat prominent spots about the size of a lentil which, as a rule, grow pale upon pressure; some of these were truly haemorrhagic. Dr Lowson assured me that they were caused by mosquitoes, and the patients said so too. I asked several sick Japanese whether the mosquito bites caused such circumcised, round reddish spots, before being taken sick. They all answered my question in the negative, and wondered themselves that, after they were taken sick by the pest, all mosquito bites made red spots.'

Convalescing, already dreaming of home, Aoyama had settled for the closest solution to hand. There was no experimental follow-up, no control groups for comparison, but then the scientist – coming round from a two-week plague coma – can have been in no shape to attempt further research. It was thus that he limped home to Tokyo, his notebook filled with supposition and half-truth, incomplete data and bold conclusion, to be greeted as a national hero.

*

TO SCIENTISTS ACROSS the world, plague in Hong Kong was a drama that – through journals and newspaper reports, letters from colleagues and grapevine murmurs – became increasingly gripping as the epidemic wore on. The fullest record, the most avid week-by-week commentary, came from the London-based weekly *Lancet*, and subscribers from Rio de Janeiro to San Francisco, Edinburgh to Bombay, would have eagerly followed events and awaited news of breaththrough, piecing together clues to the rivalry between Kitasato and Yersin, even as they worried over the possibility of plague splintering out from Asia and reaching their own territories.

To begin with, the tone of the *Lancet* dispatches was strangely distanced, even a little aloof. Such an outbreak, they seemed to imply, was the manifest outcome of a primitive way of life, too-basic hygiene, and ignorance typical of the 'oriental'. 'The disorder,' stated a report in the 16 June issue, 'is said to be "bubonic plague", but as yet little is known beyond the fact that a most serious epidemic has occurred.' Only reluctantly – stressing that 'among an ignorant and superstitious population it is natural to attribute the sudden appearance of an epidemic and fatal disease to plague' – was it admitted that the disease bore 'a remarkable resemblance to the plague which, some 230 years before, visited London, and of which Defoe has left us such a graphic account'.

A week on, however, all equivocation had disappeared, though the *Lancet*'s tone of lofty distance was zealously maintained: the outbreak was now 'oriental plague', not 'bubonic plague', whose medieval European history was then described in all its bloody detail. The spread of contagion – less than an hour, according to Boccaccio – was spelled out, and the symptoms lingered over with an indecorous degree of relish. 'Small black pustules [were] distributed over the whole skin of the body'; 'many died . . .

through vomiting blood'; the term 'Black Death [came] from the appearance of the skin after death'. The comparison between the London of 1665 – when houses were 'low, unventilated and undrained', and 'bulls, oxen, hogs and other gross creatures were slaughtered in the street' – and the 'native quarter of Hong Kong where the coolies congregate and live' was self-evident. There was, however, occasion for hope, reported the *Lancet* on 23 June: a telegraph from Hong Kong – sent by James Lowson – 'informs us that Professor Kitasato of Tokio [sic], late assistant of Professor Koch's laboratory in Berlin, has succeeded in discovering the bacillus of the plague'.

Two weeks later, on 7 July, the tentative reception of Kitasato's news had become unrestrained affirmation. Quoting 'our correspondent in Hong Kong' – again, most likely Lowson – the *Lancet* editorial went on to state that 'little doubt is any longer entertained by scientific opinion in China as to the importance of the discovery by Professor Kitasato'. News of 'other announcements of similar researches' – reported a month later, on 4 August – was treated derisively, almost as a source of comedy. Yersin's name was even misspelt – as 'Versin' – and his motivation questioned. He was noted, tongue-in-cheek, as having 'discovered another bacillus, which he, too, claims to be the essential cause of the disease; and others, equally anxious to discover something, have swelled the list, so that, as our correspondent says, "the varieties of plague bacilli now outnumber the leaves in Vallombrosa" '.

History, however, records no such others: the exaggeration here bears Lowson's stamp. Unquestioningly repeating Lowson's libellous asides, the journal returned to the one still point, the sole certainty: Kitasato. 'The name of Kitasato is a guarantee of accuracy in observation and care in research, and when the opportunity is given for the review of his work it will probably be found to meet the severest tests.' Set against such a colossus, the 'local *savants* keen on discovering a specific bacillus' – the derogatory French usage making this a deliberate maligning of Yersin, the only French bacteriologist at work in Hong Kong – could be comfortably dismissed, 'their' research no more threatening to Kitasato's hegemony than the posturings of a precocious child.

And yet, despite the apparent certainty – the insistence that only Kitasato was to be taken seriously – a note of confusion began to infiltrate the *Lancet*. On 11 August, Yersin's initial results were printed. The disease, readers learned, took four to six days to incubate, 'and then [it] commences suddenly with loss of strength . . . death occurs in twenty-four hours, or it may be delayed until the fourth or fifth day'. The bacillus was 'abundant in the buboes . . . and very rare in the blood at the time of death'. Mice injected with the bacillus died within twenty-four hours.

A week on came the backlash. Of particular concern to the editors was that Yersin 'claims to have discovered *the* bacillus of the Chinese plague. We think there must be some misapprehension here, as Professor Kitasato is such an accurate and reliable observer that we cannot conceive that he has rushed into print without having first satisfied himself as to the accuracy of his observations and experiments.' Yet doubt, now, had reared its head: in denying that Kitasato had been precipitate, the *Lancet* was admitting that this unwelcome possibility was even worthy of consideration. To scientists across the world reading this latest update, the sudden uncertainty would have had all the weight of a whodunnit: *had* he been rushed, and if so, by whom? And why?

*

A WEEK ON FROM the Hong Kong Governor's approval of Yersin's request to conduct autopsies, the bacteriologist had managed to study some twenty-five cadavers. This was swift progress: after being so long restrained, Yersin was working as fast as he could, collapsing into his bed only when his eyes began to fail in the candlelight. The conditions were tough: based now in his hurriedly built grass hut, he would have had little protection from heat or mosquitoes, yet only a single reference to physical hardship survives.

Able now to focus more intently on his own work, Yersin found himself less preoccupied by news of Kitasato. Writing on 21 July to his friend Albert Calmette at the Pasteur Institute, he noted without obvious pique that the government 'heaps kindnesses on the Japanese . . . The Governor has offered them one of his villas for the duration of their stay; he sent a telegram to the Mikado to express his profound admiration for Kitasato's magnificent discovery.'

Yersin, for his part, viewed this 'discovery' with scorn: Kitasato's report of his findings, published in the papers the day before, was 'a long screed' whose reasoning 'would make La Palisse shudder'. To equate Kitasato with La Palisse – a late nineteenth-century writer synonymous with the purveyance of mindless platitudes – was the gravest insult Yersin could devise. 'In short,' he finished, 'it won't be difficult to do better than that.'

By now, with the newspapers filled with little else but plague, and detailed discussion of the two bacteriologists' researches, an everyday routine was becoming increasingly hard to sustain. Working in the open, with no way of barring entry to his hut, Yersin must have been an obvious target for the autograph hunter and plague tourist. Interruptions were commonplace. To Calmette he confided his mounting irritation. 'People will keep coming and annoying me by asking to see the microbe. Each day unknown "ladies" and "gentlemen" enter my house without even being announced and ask me to show them preparations and cultures.'

It was then, no doubt at least in part through a desire to escape the cascade of intrusions, that he began to intersperse his laboratory research with lone, exploratory journeys through the worst-hit parts of Hong Kong. One can picture him, notebook in hand, sketching and scribbling, standing at street corners trying to square what he was seeing with what he already knew. Early on, he was struck by the inadequacies of the drainage system: in Taipingshan, he noticed, a new labyrinth of drains had been installed before this same neighbourhood became the crucible of plague, and so he walked the now-deserted streets, hunting for clues. Could the sewers, he wondered, have actually triggered the outbreak? 'The system,' he wrote to the French Governor-General of Indochina, 'seems defective . . . One cannot understand why in Hong Kong there are two very distinct sorts of drains: one wide and well conditioned for draining rainwater; the other narrow, continually getting blocked, for household water and household waste.' The combination of inadequate waste-disposal and the physical congestion of the area made it 'easy to understand the ravages which an epidemic can make when it takes hold on such territory and the difficulty that there must be in checking its progress'.

Gradually, he began to hone his powers of deduction.

Unlike Kitasato – whose writings contain only scanty descriptions of goings-on outside the laboratory, and for whom the worlds of science and everyday life appear to have existed in parallel, seldom converging – Yersin was drawn to the everyday, to the clues that lay all around him. Rats, he noted, were dying 'en masse'; and experiments proved that they, too, were victims of plague. By mid July, he alone among all the scientific community was convinced that 'rats are certainly the principal propagators of the epidemic', although their exact role eluded him. The drains, he postulated, may have been the link: 'These animals live in drains where they maintain the illness in its sporadic state. It is impossible to disinfect or to chase them out of there, since the pipes are too narrow.'

He was halfway there, tantalizingly close. All around were false leads, red herrings, chief among them the fact that 'the European population has been relatively little touched by the plague. Why? Because it lives in hygienic conditions which are far superior to those of the Chinese. I know several European houses where rats have died in great numbers and where, nonetheless, no one has caught plague. That is because people always took care to remove the corpses and to disinfect thoroughly.'

Too quick to take his eye off the rat as a possible carrier of plague, Yersin, writing again to the Governor-General, cast around for other possible culprits. Why not the common fly? he suggested. 'I have experiments which prove that they can die from this disease. It is easily understood that a fly which has landed on the corpse of a plague rat and which then walks on the bare leg of a Chinese man, where there are very often abrasions and ulcers, could very easily transmit the disease to him.'

'Direct contagion' also seemed 'very likely'. However, this theory, like so much else, left him isolated. 'Several Hong Kong doctors' – almost certainly James Lowson and his entourage – opposed him. Undeterred, Yersin proceeded to devise an experiment to prove his thesis. Into the same container he placed a healthy mouse and a second into which he'd injected concentrated plague suspension. He repeated the experiment several times and the results, he claimed, were not only conclusive – 'I have often seen both animals die of plague' – but indicative of the wider picture. 'The Chinese who live crammed in narrow spaces are in the same position as my mice. And the other day I saw five Chinese who slept in a sort of narrow cellar catch the illness one after the other.'

For the first time, Yersin was stumbling. His argument was incomplete: if plague was contagious, as he claimed, what was the method of transmission? That question, at least for the moment, remained unanswered.

*

SOME THIRTEEN YEARS LATER, with the flea–rat–man axis by now firmly accepted, the authorities in San Francisco – fighting to repair roads, hospitals and schools in the wake of earthquake and fire – found themselves facing their second outbreak of plague. This time, however, the path before them was clear, the enemy known. In 1901, the city's first plague epidemic had found them riven, arguing among themselves over the mechanism of the disease, how best to contain it, even its very existence. Now, in 1907, there was no such tussle: the battle was on.

Never in its 130-year history had the city offered such a promising breeding-ground for plague. The earthquake of

18 April 1906 – measuring 8.3 on the Richter scale, making it ten times as powerful as that which tore through the metropolis in 1989 – lasted forty-seven seconds, by the end of which almost the entire downtown area lay ruined. Then came the fires: fractured gas mains and toppling chimneys triggered explosions of flame which the Fire Department, finding only broken water pipes, was unable to douse. Nothing went right: attempts at creating firebreaks by dynamiting entire city blocks only succeeded in sparking fresh fires. Seventy-two hours later, when the last blaze had finally been extinguished, four-and-a-half square miles of the city was rubble, smouldering timbers jutting from the wreckage like a broken skeleton, remains of a once-great beast. Photographs of the aftermath bring to mind post-firestorm Dresden: the outline of the streets is jagged, the top half of all buildings destroyed; items of salvaged furniture – pianos, coffee tables – stand in the street; a soldier picks his way along a pavement of strewn bricks; everywhere is smoke, rising poisonous and impenetrable into the broken sky.

Some three thousand people died that first week, and more than a hundred thousand – a third of the population – were rendered homeless, squatting in tent cities in the parks and on the burnt-out lot of Charles Croker's Nob Hill estate. Itinerant workers poured into the city, hired as emergency construction gangs. With the waste-disposal system no longer in operation, vacant downtown grids became vast, unpoliced dumps. When plague finally struck in August 1907, it was the scenario that everyone had been fearing and anticipating: the only surprise was that it had taken this long to take hold.

As the epidemic ground on, it became apparent that, for plague to be beaten, the whole city would have to be

involved, and in January 1908, with the epidemic still
showing no signs of abating, a 'citizens' committee' was
assembled: twenty-five prominent traders and businessmen
and doctors, charged with the task of convincing the rest of
the populace that they were confronting 'one of the great
malign forces of nature'. Posters were designed and signed
by every member of the committee – twelve of whom
carried the reassuring suffix MD – exhorting the public to
'Trap and Poison Rats! Obey the Sanitary Laws of the City!
Have your Premises Inspected!' The copy, set in a dizzying
variety of type sizes, seemed itself designed to engender
panic. 'The dreaded "Bubonic Plague" has reappeared in
San Francisco since the fire and is gaining ground. Should
the Plague continue to show a marked increase, San Francisco will probably be quarantined. This would be a death
blow to the industrial life of the city and would bring ruin
to our people and our homes . . . It is incumbent upon
all to wage a relentless war on the Rat.'

Churchillian rhetoric duly delivered, the citizens' committee set about the considerable task of public education.
A meeting of butchers and fruit-and-vegetable wholesalers
was called, and the tradesmen ordered to use only water-
tight metal garbage cans: butchers in particular were singled
out and instructed to abandon use of their open-topped
wooden scrap bins. The message caught on quickly: by
early February the 'sub-committee of the clergy' – a five-
man cross-denominational team of vicars and rabbis – was
issuing instructions that 'every minister of a congregation,
according to his own judgement, present from his pulpit to
his people the necessity of continuing effort in promoting
the sanitation of San Francisco'; that the same propaganda

be spelled out in 'Sunday school assemblies'; and that the churches themselves be rat-proofed.

Determination to be rid of plague – unlike Hong Kong a decade earlier – even crossed cultural boundaries. In March, the Japanese Association posted fliers demanding that all assistance be offered in the fight against the disease. 'CLEANLINESS IS THE JAPANESE NATURE' shouted the headline, above a list of 'directions for the care of the bedroom, kitchen, porch, garbage can, etc'. The first of these was straightforward – 'Kill all the rats' – though it was necessary to read as far as point nine before the helpful 'Do not kill rats with your hands' was added. Fleas should be exterminated with equal caution: 'Don't use your fingers or teeth.'

To cover the eventuality that there might exist children who did not attend Sunday school, a crew of doctors was conscripted to spread the message in the classroom. One contemporary account reported that 'the pupils evinced a lively interest in what they were told', which seems hardly surprising, since the material cunningly appealed to their baser natures, in particular the sneak that lurks inside the heart of every otherwise blameless eight-year-old. 'The rats from a neighbouring house may be dangerous to man. Therefore, uncleanly [sic] neighbours are dangerous . . . To protect life one must watch one's neighbours and report them if they are uncleanly.' But most attractive of all, one suspects, was the appeal to the pocket: 'A reward of five cents will be paid for every rat, dead or alive.' A trifling risk for a bag of boiled sweets.

Chapter Fifteen

Bombay, at the end of September 1994, was a city braced for an epidemic. It had known such before: in 1896, plague hit Bombay harbour from Hong Kong, and the disease drilled through India, killing some ten million over the next decade. Now, however, the threat was coming not from the sea, but inland, from the rotten and poisonous metropolis of Surat some two hundred kilometres to the north.

Within hours of the first Surat plague deaths, and with intelligence coming fast about the numbers fleeing by road and train, the Bombay health department ordered the immediate setting-up of surveillance posts. Doctors with clipboards and bags of diagnostic equipment waited on station platforms, at bus stops and checkpoints along the highway. Cars with the Surat suffix – GJ5 – were pulled over and searched, the occupants interrogated and ordered to drive straight to the Kasturba Infectious Diseases Hospital. In the still moments before the whirlwind, there was a surreal sense of having been here before: another time, with different people, but the same story.

A more recent traveller, navigating the choked streets of Bombay – seeing the free-for-all at traffic lights; the man asleep on the pavement at ten in the morning, scarlet flower caught in his moustache; the rat leaping the gully between

two high buildings – could easily have imagined the chaos
should disease strike here. As in Hong Kong in 1894, the
conditions were perfect: overcrowding, dirt, inadequate
drainage, unclean water, ignorance and worse.

The Bombay Hospital was cross-hatched with rickety
bamboo scaffolding; Dr Jehangir Sorabjee, the hospital's
infectious diseases specialist, smiled and gave a tiny shrug
as a chunk of concrete fell past the window. News of the
1994 outbreak in Surat had reached him, he said, from a
doctor friend.

'He rang up and said he was getting a whole stream of
patients from Surat saying they were evacuating the city
because plague had broken out. He wanted to know what
medicines he should be giving them, what the symptoms
were. I was shocked to hear of this, but within hours there
it was on the news. I was at the Kasturba Hospital at the
time and we convened a meeting and decided to discharge
all patients and prepare for a really big outbreak. People
arriving from Surat were asked to come in for testing. It
was a very strange experience – people wandering the corridors of the hospital dressed in surgical gear with their heads
covered in muslin cloths, tiny slits for their eyes. It felt like
the Martians had landed.'

Sorabjee and colleagues decided to test for plague using
slides and microscopes; if they couldn't find the bacillus,
they'd refuse to confirm any patient as plague-positive. Elsewhere, however, different diagnostic procedures were used,
and doctors opting for serological testing – which gauges
the presence and volume of antibodies in the blood of
an infected person, deducing from this the exact disease
responsible – came up with dramatic positive results. Where

Sorabjee's bacteriological testing had drawn a blank, the
serum experiments screamed danger.

So what was going on? In Surat, the medical superintendent of the city's biggest hospital had insisted the disease
had indeed been plague, and subsequent work by the
Atlanta-based Center for Communicable Diseases had confirmed this. Yet here was Sorabjee, eminent disease specialist
and a man with no obvious special interest, maintaining
the opposite. Clearly plague, of all diseases, was the very
last any health professional would wish on his country: as
Sorabjee confessed, even overseas doctors began cancelling
trips to India. He shook his head. 'One of my colleagues
had organized the world congress on cancer-related diseases
at that time in New Delhi, and forty per cent of his delegates
cried off.' Even among the most worldly medics, it seemed,
mention of plague still summoned up the barbarous Middle
Ages.

Among the politicians, however, the same fears assumed
more manipulative, paranoid form: doctors, Sorabjee
admitted, were under constant pressure 'to suppress the
incidence of certain communicable diseases. Take cholera.
There are cases all through the year, but because of the
worry about international maritime regulations they try and
get us to record it as something else – gastro-enteritis, for
instance. Cholera reported in Bombay – like plague – would
have tremendous economic implications. People would
cancel holidays, tourism would collapse.'

He weaved, avoiding giving direct answers, since to have
done so, one imagined, would have meant admitting not
only to a schism in the country's medical establishment, but
also impugning the integrity of colleagues with whom he

could not agree. He leant across the desk, pressed his palms together.

'Once,' he smiled, seeming more than ever the soothing GP, 'I remember walking with Mother Teresa through the slums of Bombay. These were just typical areas, the way most people live, but even she was shocked. She said, "I've seen slums in Calcutta, but never as bad as this." She was not a lady who was easy to shock, and the overcrowding is just getting worse. The question to ask of 1994 is not whether plague occurred at all but why it hasn't appeared more often.'

*

NIGHT, AND MOHANLAL was travelling north. This, the Ahmedabad Janata Express, was the third train he'd attempted to board, and in his growing desperation he'd abandoned every last trace of politeness and clawed and punched his way on. Even by normal Indian standards – where trains are often so crowded grown men sit on each other's knees, squat in the luggage racks, down the steps and along all passageways – this was farcically cramped. For ten minutes at least, he'd been hanging on to the doorjamb, the door swinging open behind him, track thundering by underneath. Then finally, and only by striking at others' ankles till they yelped and moved, he had managed to move inside enough to secure the door behind him.

Once inside, he found it impossible to get anyone to answer him. Whenever he spoke, all would turn their faces away, covering their mouths. There were other Suratis in this carriage, but they'd been barricaded into one corner, and were being similarly blocked. The windows were all open, and the through-blast blew dust and scraps of paper

over people's heads. A polystyrene cup came spinning
through the air and was sucked out of a window on the
other side of the carriage. In the press of bodies, he felt his
feet lift off the floor. Silently, he prayed for the structure of
the train, for the rivets and sheet steel to hold firm.

Compared with the smell and heat and crush inside,
the view from the window seemed paradisaical. Normally,
he'd have been happy to be inside, rather than standing
under a naked sun in a landscape baked dry as biscuit, but
today the solitary figures in the fields seemed unbearably
fortunate. A man – shoeless, carrying two bulging plastic
bags – strolled past bushes pale with dust, towards a mud-
brick house. He stopped at the threshold, turned towards
the train and waved. No one waved back.

At the first stop north of Surat, a hefty man with a neck
too big for his shirt collar threatened to throw Mohanlal
from the train. Mohanlal turned away, knowing that any
response would be read as provocation. The man began
shouting. 'You! Get off this train!' Mohanlal felt a hand on
his shoulder, but he knew the crowd was too tightly packed
to force him off, however much they might have wanted to.
After what seemed an age he heard the couplings clank and
the platform began to inch away from them.

He was aware of the risks of being fingered as a fleeing
Surati, and was determined to hold on to his place on the
train. Anand – where he was sure Hetal would have gone
– was still some three hours off, and he knew that if he
was ejected before that he risked being stoned or worse by
fearful territorial villagers. Already, he'd heard, a bus loaded
with diamond workers had been pelted with rocks as it
entered Banaskantha district. In a Rajkot village, residents
had been standing at entry points with long bamboo

lathis, fending off all outsiders: a self-appointed vigilante posse, the more terrifying for being outside the law. Alone, Mohanlal knew, he'd make an easy target.

The further they travelled from Surat, the quieter and less populous the stations became. At a small town some way south of Vadodara five people got out, and Mohanlal found a seat arm against which to rest. He felt dazed; his brain was fogged by the heat. On the platform he noticed a prosthetic leg lying abandoned, and gazed at it blankly without wondering how it had got there. It was as if curiosity, normally his dominant trait, had died as fear had risen: with his wife and daughter still unaccounted for, he found it impossible to focus on anything else. Shop signs that normally would have caused a wry smile – 'Family Fashion Point. Free Compliment on Purchase!' – now barely registered.

Though not a religious man, he found himself praying as the train approached Anand, mumbling incantations for the safety of his family. He had a good idea of the route Hetal would have taken, and could picture the long straight track through the fields that led from town to the village and the smallholding of his parents-in-law. What he did not know was what might have lain in wait for them along the way: the vigilantes out patrolling for plague refugees; others, for whom the appearance of any outsider could prove the fuse for violence, alert for any excuse to stir up suspicion between Muslim and Hindu. These days, it seemed, it took so little to rouse hatred: the riots of 1992, the burning of temples and mosques: so many reasons not to believe, if this was the outcome of religious fervour. Yet still he prayed.

*

FOR INDIA, the Surat plague of September and October 1994 swiftly became a test of nationhood, of its effectiveness and strength: how, with every overseas government watching and assessing, would the subcontinent move to stamp out disease? At airports, harbours and railway stations, the campaign was immediate, and visible to the point of high comedy: aeroplanes were not only fumigated but searched by white-gloved technicians for the presence of rats, and one can picture them on their hands and knees in the airless, sweltering baggage holds, their ears to the metalwork, alert for the telltale scritch-scritch of rodents.

In Surat, on 29 September, the plague suspects who had fled barefoot and breathless from the New Civil Hospital were warned by the district magistrate – in all newspapers and on every available radio bulletin – that unless they returned within twenty-four hours they faced 'penal action'. To ratchet up the level of terror, a quivering public was then informed that two 'rapid action force' teams had been dispatched to track down the lawbreakers. None were ever found, but the lightning legislation did not end there: anyone discovered expectorating in a public place faced immediate arrest.

For more than a month, schools remained closed, food vendors' pitches lay empty. People ventured out of doors only when their larders were bare, and then with their faces covered, heads down. Yet this picture of desolation and fear did not apply throughout the city, for Surat is above all a commercial centre, and there were some for whom the lure of profit overshadowed everything else. At Hare Krishna Export, a six-floor steel-and-glass temple to the diamond industry, it became clear for the first time that this city, which had done nothing to prevent a great many from living lives of disease and squalor in their soft-floored polythene shacks, was also the comfortable home to a handful of very rich men.

The boss sat behind a desk of polished glass, the legs like fluted, gold-leafed Doric columns. Behind him was a painting so garish it was hard to look at anything else: a scene from an Elysian Eden, with embossed, silvery waterfalls and sunlight that splintered golden through the clouds.

This was the second floor, possibly the third: it was easy to lose one's bearings during the security checks, the body searches, the elevator that took for ever, the uniformed guards that seemed to have been posted on every corner. A brief tour of the offices had revealed floor upon floor of workers, silent and assiduous as drones. On one level, men and women had sat silently peering through magnifying glasses at diamonds, some pinprick-tiny. On another, hotter level, it was difficult to focus over the whine and hammer of polishing machines. Measuring the diamonds – before they were marked and cut – took place on computer, and the operator spun and calibrated the stone, then lifted it off its measuring wheel and drew black lines across its rough outer edge where the cutter – on yet another floor – would reveal its final shape.

The company, said the boss, stroking his phone in its cradle, employed two thousand people across five cities. 'In Surat alone, there are between five and six hundred diamond companies. This is diamond city.'

Diamond-cutting was Surat's most profitable industry, a middle link in a chain of supply and demand that began with dealers in Belgium and ended with jewellers in Manhattan and Hong Kong. Such was the commitment of the diamond operatives that, during the outbreak of plague,

not one employee fled. 'At Hare Krishna Export, nobody
went anywhere. We are businessmen. We have a business
to run.'

*

THE PLAGUE IN SURAT, it was becoming clear, was but a
corner of a much broader canvas, and diamond-cutting,
just as much as the manifest degradation of the Ved Road
slums, was a part. In a healthier society, the profits from
such businesses would have been harnessed – even if only
to a modest degree – and spent on street-cleaning, welfare
programmes, low-cost housing. But not in Surat. From
the earliest years of its growth as an industrial centre,
Surat – more than any other Indian city – had resisted
direct taxation, and the resulting lack of funding had
hastened decay and epidemic. As early as the 1890s, sanitation experts were advising that underground drainage should
be introduced as a matter of urgency, but – despite an early
twentieth-century death-from-epidemic rate of some ninety
per thousand – such a system was not built until 1956.
Throughout Surat's inglorious history, any suggestion of
raised taxes had met with strikes and riots: a proposed
income tax in 1890 provoked a citywide business closedown;
a tax on businesses in 1878 incited several days of rioting.
The political community – still nascent throughout India –
was in Surat close to embryonic. From builders came the
same, wearingly familiar story: that construction could only
begin once the appropriate government officers had been
paid off, after underworld heavies had been hired for protection. The rich, it was clear, did not depend upon the sewage
system, the telephone network or the public hospitals: they

paid for their own, and saw little need to contribute to anyone else's.

*

IT WAS DAWN when Mohanlal's train pulled into Anand. He'd not slept, but at least the train was less crowded now, and he'd been able to wrestle himself a corner of step to sit on. His heart was beating erratically: it felt like an animal, a small bird, struggling to escape its cage. With no warning, as the landscape turned from trees to burned scrub, the sun came blinding through the window. There was coughing all up the carriage: those who'd managed to sleep startled suddenly awake.

Deprived of food, water and sleep, he found his consciousness was playing tricks on him: electrically alert one moment, seemingly drugged the next. With little money, he walked through the centre of Anand, past chai sellers boiling up their first brew, waking sleeping dogs with the dust he kicked up. He rode two buses, barely having enough strength to ask the driver his destination, until the shanties of the outskirts became dusty fields and the wayside emptied of people, until only the occasional cow stopped to watch them pass. At a crossroads, the driver shouted back to Mohanlal: the bus was returning to Anand; from here he was on his own.

It felt like years since he'd been this way, though his last visit with Hetal to her parents' village could not have been more than six months ago. He leant against a tree, barely cooler in the shade, and tried to remember the turn-off, or any distinguishing features in a landscape that seemed now to him to be utterly devoid of landmarks, flat and stripped of vegetation, just the occasional goat tethered to a bony tree.

His shoes had started to rub, and he took them off. For a while, his mind in neutral, he walked on in his socks until a boy, passing on a bicycle, glanced at his feet and laughed. In that moment, the butt of the most innocent, childlike joke, he felt himself alone as never before. Fear and homesickness rose like bile in his throat. Reaching the house, he sat down against a wall, laid his head back and closed his eyes.

He awoke sweating and uneasy. He opened his eyes, but the sun was high now and his vision was blurred, tinged pale blue, as if chlorine-affected. He could see there were figures standing in front of him: a small child, two adults, though they remained in silhouette. He tried to stand, but felt his legs go weak under him, and so remained on the ground. He shaded his eyes from the sun, tried to breathe normally.

'What are you doing here?' It was a male voice, suspicious.

Mohanlal, his throat suddenly dry as sand, whispered the name of the village where he was headed. 'Some water?' he added, barely getting the words out. 'I am thirsty.'

'Why are you going there? You have no car, no buses come this way. It will take you hours.'

'My wife,' Mohanlal said, suddenly close to tears again. 'She is there. My daughter too.' He could see their features more clearly now: the dot of sandalwood paste on the woman's forehead glistening scarlet; a wire-and-cork toy car that the little boy was clutching so tight it seemed he was worried for its safety.

The man whispered something to the woman, and they both took a pace backwards, pulling the boy with them.

'Get out of here,' the man grunted.

'But . . .' Mohanlal began to protest, but he stopped mid-sentence, realizing words were useless. The man was holding up a stick now, angled towards Mohanlal's chest as he struggled to his feet.

'Be gone,' the man said. 'You come back this way, and I kill you.'

*

To PROFESSOR Shibasaburo Kitasato, convinced that the race was his, that he was the first scientist to have discovered the bacillus that caused bubonic plague, the persistence of Dr Alexandre Yersin must have seemed pointless, even impudent. Kitasato paused in his work, surrounded by the white coats of his research team, and glanced from his window. From Kennedy Town plague hospital, where he had established his laboratory, it was but three hundred yards across a strip of trampled mud to Yersin's modest *paillotte* and the more substantial straw-and-wood longhouse now serving as overflow plague ward. To Kitasato, Yersin's accommodation would have seemed ridiculous: no serious scientist would ever have settled for such pitiable conditions.

In mid-July governor Sir William Robinson asked Kitasato for a research update that he could send to the British Colonial Secretary, the Marquess of Ripon, in London. To have been able to dispatch a sample of heavyweight science signed by the peerless Kitasato would, he'd have felt, go a long way towards silencing his increasingly restless superiors, whose telegrams to Hong Kong had recently taken on an impatient air. Once they read of Kitasato's work, they would have no cause to doubt that Robinson had recruited the best, for Kitasato's name was as much a brand as that of Pasteur, or Koch: a guarantee of quality.

Kitasato rose to the commission in a prose style that seems self-consciously and uncharacteristically casual. He addressed the British government as he might have a colleague; his confidence was clearly boundless; he felt unimpeachable, expansive. 'This recent outbreak,' he remarked, 'has given us the opportunity for studying this disease – a cause of mystery for centuries – with the means which modern science places in our hands.' He spoke of the autopsies carried out, the observations made, and then laid out his 'proof', a three-point argument which, he'd have felt, rendered his position unassailable.

First, the bacillus he claimed to have discovered was present only in the buboes, blood and internal organs of plague patients. Second, it was not found in any other infectious disease and was, therefore, unique to plague. Third, it induced in animals symptoms identical to those observed in humans. His conclusion left no room for doubt. 'This Bacillus is the cause of the disease known as bubonic plague, therefore the bubonic plague is an infectious disease produced by a specific bacillus.'

Nor did he stop there. Mindful no doubt of the preju-dices of his readers, of the disinclination of the bureaucratic classes to read purely of science – however stunning the breakthrough – he then addressed himself to the practical. Experiments in which he'd managed to destroy the bacillus, both by exposing it to direct sunlight and by boiling it, demonstrated beyond doubt the measures necessary to keep it at bay: 'General hygiene, good drainage, perfect water supply, cleanliness in dwelling houses, and cleanliness in the

streets'. Taipingshan – which fell short in every category –
was 'a suitable hunting-ground for the Plague Bacillus'.

The next step for Kitasato – as for Yersin – was to
investigate conceivable routes of contagion; whether it was
possible to develop the disease through contact with an
animal, insect or another person; or whether plague was,
rather, a disease of the soil, and that exposure to 'bad' earth
could lead to infection.

The latter theory dated to ancient times and – in the
Hong Kong of 1894 as in the Mediterranean basin of
the first century BC – was often allied to talk of poisoned
air. First propounded by Hippocrates, the concept that
meteorological conditions affected human health had
proved impressively durable. Scientific thinkers as early as
Jerome Fracastor – in his 1546 *De Contagione* – had proposed
a mechanism of infection whereby tissues of the body were
invaded by invisible particles. At the end of the nineteenth
century, it was this school of thought – pathogenic air and
corrupted earth – that still commanded most respect.

Yersin and Kitasato would have kept up to date with
the latest scientific papers, and so would have been aware
of the weight of opinion arguing against plague as a disease
that could only be caught from other humans or animals.
As late as 1890, the respected British medical historian
Charles Creighton was claiming that it was, in fact, a soil-
borne offshoot of typhus: 'When ordinary typhus has passed
into a soil poison, by aggravation of conditions, as in the
experience of Arab encampments in North Africa [a reference to the Tunisian outbreak of 1874], it has become at
the same time bubonic fever, or, approximately plague
proper.' In Hong Kong itself, the medical establishment, led
by government bacteriologist William Hunter, was working

on a theory of infected food. Hunter claimed to have discovered plague bacilli in rice, in particular the low-grade
grain used by the poorest Chinese; this, he said, had been
infected by flies, which in turn had carried the bacillus from
the diseased excreta of plague rats. He was pointing in the
right direction, but no more.

Over the coming weeks, as July lengthened into August
and the evacuation and sluice-through of Taipingshan had
caused the rate of infection to begin to ease off, Yersin
and Kitasato – under orders from the government – found
themselves in the same part of the island, exploring a similar
field of possibility. Their investigations took place in Taipingshan, which was now being targeted for demolition by a
government anxious to be seen to be taking decisive action.
Taipingshan was a compact area – just ten acres, in which
384 houses had been shoehorned – and was also, by July,
close to deserted. A team of Kitasato's size – six scientists,
no doubt trailing a retinue of government doctors – would
have been hard to miss as it gathered in the street with
trays of sterile containers and loud talk, each competing for
the attention of Kitasato, master of ceremonies.

By contrast, Yersin, the lone researcher, would have
been close to invisible. In his bulletin of 4 August to the
Indochinese Governor-General, he explains that, like Kitasato, he had been asked by the Hong Kong government
some three weeks earlier to 'examine the soil of houses
where there have been plague cases in order to find out
whether or not they contained the germs of the illness'.
His language – 'I sent myself to Taipingshan' – seems
determinedly unselfconscious for, if the popular infection
theories were correct, he was about to enter the most contagious area. And yet there is no hint of fear, nor any sense

that he even took precautions: his focus was solely on the work ahead.

A photograph pasted into the back of the manuscript folio of '*Voyage à Hong Kong au Sujet de la Peste*' pictures the plague streets themselves. It is taken from low down, as if Yersin, to emphasize the gradient that climbs away from him, had fallen to his knees, camera at an angle close to thirty, forty degrees. The viewer thus stands at this cross-street – a sign high up on a house corner says 'Caine Lane', now a sweeping asphalt curve between high glass-faced apartment buildings, then the heart of the plague district – and everywhere is rubble, heaps of smashed and splintered wood. Low down on the walls are peeling posters.

Ahead, between buildings from which shutters hang from broken hinges, climbs a narrow street, every twenty yards another steep bank of steps. From the faded print it is hard to make out where the street ends, whether it peters out into scrub or is blocked by another cross-street. Outside every door there are mounds of charred debris: what remained after the soldiers threw out every last item of furniture and bedding from the houses, and then set the torch to them. It is a scene which seems only possible in monochrome, as if colour, faced with such desolation and abandonment, would simply dissolve.

Then Yersin packed away his camera and began to walk up the street. He carried with him a steel tin, a small trowel, notebook, pencil. At the top of the first flight of steps he stopped and looked around, wondering which house to start with. All were abandoned: from each dwelling, he had been told, plague dead had been carried. The nearest door offered no chance of entry, having been rough-nailed shut; the entrances to others had been rendered near-impassable by rubble and broken timber. However, two houses on, he could see a door swinging open. There were smashed chairs outside, the charred ribs of a bed-frame, and he stepped gingerly through the debris. A dog, standing alone at the top of the street, watched him, head on one side.

He stood for a while at the doorway, letting his eyes adjust to the darkness inside. Being mid-terrace, the house had no side windows; peering in, he could see none at the back either. He took a step forward, turned the corner, and hammered with the heel of his hand at the shutter that was cutting out the light from the street. When it finally gave, he saw that he was standing on a floor of uneven mud; when he moved he left deep footprints. Despite the open window and door, there was a powerful and disagreeable smell. He began to hunt for a simile, for the stench reminded him of something, maybe the belch of methane as a scalpel cuts into a week-old corpse, but the search defeated him: the smell was too complex, too aged and layered, to be so easily pinned down.

He felt dampness on his shoulder. He stepped back. Something was dripping from the floor above, coming through the floorboards. It fell not like water, in bright tiny bulbs, but in long gloopy tendrils. The colour – red-streaked yellow, like phlegm flecked with blood – repulsed him, for it brought to mind the gleety discharge exuded by eyes and other wet tissue at the time of death. His feet were starting to feel cold, and he knew that mud had already penetrated his shoe leather.

He wondered where to conduct his dig. Anywhere fairly central – away from the most inaccessible corners – would, he guessed, be suitable, but first, out of curiosity, and since he was starting to question how anyone, let alone the typical extended Chinese family of twenty or thirty, could ever happily inhabit such a confined and unpromising space, he climbed the stairs. The steps were narrow, and creaked alarmingly; when he touched the wall for balance, his hand came away dark with soot.

On the first floor, as at ground level, there was a single window, but this was only of use to the central section of the room. The space had been divided into three cubicles about twelve feet square, each of which, he knew, would have served as the living space for a family of five or six. He shook his head, beyond astonishment, and then he spotted the source of the dripping – a decaying piece of meat, black with flies, weeping dark ooze into the surrounding floorboards. He turned for the stairs again, in a hurry now, and slipped near the bottom, his elbow grazed black against the wall.

His trowel dug easily into the floor: he'd imagined it being a vigorous work of excavation, through hard-packed earth, but it crumbled with an ease that made him ponder again the reality of living in such conditions: in near-darkness, with little privacy, upon an unsealed floor. With each fresh trowelful of dirt, it seemed more and more plausible that the earth itself did indeed harbour infection: he filled his tin as quickly as he could and exited into the daylight, breathing deeply, filling his lungs with morning air that now felt unusually, blessedly sweet.

*

FOR KITASATO, THE IDEA that the very soil might be a plague reservoir seemed only logical. During his seven years in Robert Koch's Berlin laboratory, Kitasato had been decisively influenced by his mentor's work on the relationship between soil and disease, in particular his anthrax research, which had demonstrated how anthrax spores could lie dormant for many years before triggering a fresh outbreak. He needed little persuasion to start from the assumption that plague propagated in a similar way.

Not for the first time, he seems like a man in a headlong hurry, overtaken by the speed of events, rushed – perhaps by the constant shadow of Yersin, quietly persistent, impossible to fluster – into errant conclusions. The mention of anthrax is there from the very start: in the report he wrote for the Hong Kong Governor at the beginning of July he was claiming that bacteriology had pinpointed 'only two micro-organisms . . . found in human blood . . . the bacillus of anthrax and the spirochaetae of relapsing fever' that produced infectious diseases in humans. The connection between anthrax and plague, he believed, was intimate: examining the way the body tissues of his laboratory animals were affected at the site of injection, he remarked that the changes were 'very similar to those found in anthrax'. So, over the coming weeks, he scoured his soil samples for the spores he was sure he would find.

For the anxious resident of colonial Hong Kong, living in self-imposed quarantine on an island bereft of the usual attractions, the news from the plague front was at best perplexing, at worst suggestive of an epidemic beyond anyone's control or understanding. While extensive coverage was given to the endeavours and rivalry of Kitasato and Yersin, equal prominence was granted both to the Chinese theories of plague transmission and to the conflicting work of senior Hong Kong doctors. Agreement seemed impossible: according to the Chinese, plague – like some kind of putrescent gas – seeped from the soil and began its spread by attacking first those animals that lived closest to the ground, before moving upwards and infecting larger animals: from rats, thus, to chickens, goats, cows and humans. To local European doctors such as Dr James Cantlie, such theories were no more than superstition – 'native popular belief' – though he had little better to offer. In the kind of convoluted language that could have come straight from a stumbling medieval medic, Cantlie argued that 'the miasma of infection seems to be soil-produced, and to flourish in filth . . . the disease is miasmatic-contagious'.

*

UNLIKE KITASATO, Yersin – carrying his first soil samples – returned to his laboratory highly sceptical, and again it was this proper caution that raised him above his precipitate rival. Writing to Albert Calmette in Paris, Yersin's lack of conviction was clear. 'Between ourselves, I have a feeling that I am embarking on this research believing that I will find nothing.'

Back in his *paillotte*, sitting at the rough trestle that served as his main workbench, hoping that at this of all moments he would not have to fend off the idle inquiries of another party of plague tourists, Yersin opened his sample tin. The smell – fainter now, neutralized a little by its isolation and containment – struck him immediately, and transported him in an instant to the sulphurous interior of the house from which he'd just returned. He turned away, coughed, took a deep breath and, with his tweezers, lifted out a crumb of the black earth. This he dropped into pre-prepared beef-broth, a culture in which the bacillus would thrive and multiply, and thus remain available for experiment. Finally, he dipped a length of platinum into the broth and pushed this into a tube of jelly. Then he waited.

He came back to his experiment expecting nothing, and there can be no mistaking the astonishment in his note to Calmette. Against every prediction, he found 'several plague colonies and another foreign microbe!!!' although – as he was swift to explain – this did not prove either the theories of the Chinese or the wayward postulations of the likes of Kitasato and Cantlie. 'I think the bacillus is attenuated [weakened, and therefore lacking potency] and today I am going to make some injections just to be sure of it.' However unlikely it seemed that infected soil was the main reservoir of plague, there was now a chink of doubt. Only if his laboratory animals survived the injections, would he be able to rule it out.

Chapter Sixteen

CLOSE UP, SECONDS FROM DEATH, *Rattus rattus,* black rat, seemed pitiable, toylike, too fineboned to be facing such a mechanical, heartless end. Its fur looked soft as rabbits' ears; its belly, as it attempted a last-minute corkscrew for freedom, was unexpectedly, touchingly pale. It had tiny hands – too human to be truly claws – with fingers agile as a monkey's. Its mouth was minutely pursed, its nose a blur of motion. The hands that gripped it – stretched shiny against the animal's matt lustre, rubbered in surgical gloves the colour of ivory – were bigger, each one, than the rat's entire length. They pressed down, pincering the rat belly-down against the yellow plastic until its legs, like a newborn baby's, were splayed flat, and its fingers grabbed at air. The glove holding the hips pushed hard, knuckles white through the latex, and the other hand began to prise away. For a moment, the rat's back looked like it might extend infinitely, and then came the snap: a point marked in time, like the crack of a twig underfoot: stillness followed.

Flipped on its back, the corpse was worked over with a bristle brush, the fur ground forward, against the grain. The hairs stood on end, and the pink of the skin was just discernible: a glow, like light through gauze. The rat had stopped moving; its marble-black eyes bulged; the brush was accumulating a downy fuzz. Under the animal's chin a cluster of dark specks danced to life, and another latexed hand entered the wide bowl, this one holding a pencil-thin glass tube. 'There! There! There!' yipped a voice. Fingers squeezed a suction bulb; the fleas were vacuumed clear.

Three feet away, surrounded by gape-mouthed children with snailtrack snot and clothes shiny with matted dirt, a woman in navy overalls and black rubber boots lifted the rat onto a chipboard slab. She, like the first two, the exterminators, was a local Malgache, and she worked with the same air of practised determination. She pressured the rat flat on its back, and now its incisors were visible: nicotine yellow, perfectly aligned, a miracle of miniature engineering. She forced the limbs wide, and drove long pins through its palms and then picked up the scalpel and drew a scarlet line from sternum to belly. She looped out the heart and let the blood drip on to a sheet of paper – six drops, soaking into six numbered circles. Looking closer, lifting out the innards with tweezers, she remarked that this was a female, in early pregnancy: seven embryos, no bigger than rice grains, were connected to each other by translucent filament.

If one overlooked the jeep from the Pasteur Institute in Antananarivo, the rat technicians and the scientists, this could have been any central Malagasy village, on any dry-heat April day. Zebu cattle were sniffing the earth in an enclosure; rice lay drying on huge raffia mats; from the top windows of red-mud houses smoke drifted, disappearing into cerulean blue. Framed by a camera, the sickly child edited out, this was a scene to quicken the pulse of any jaded Westerner: here was the simple life, pure and unadorned and close to beauty. And yet, the rats. Always the rats.

*

PLAGUE FIRST HIT Madagascar in 1898 – direct from Hong Kong, by way of Bombay, another staging post in the third pandemic as the disease, rampant, leapt continents and oceans, establishing strongholds in territory where it was hitherto unknown. In this, Madagascar was not remarkable. What was, however, and what was triggering such anxious activity from bacteriologists and researchers at the start of the twenty-first century, was that – after some five decades of quiescence – plague was back. Worse, it had returned not just in quantity but sporting new and alarming varieties. In 1995, in the southern highlands, scientists had isolated a strain of the bacillus resistant to all the main antibiotics used to treat plague. Since then, other antibiotic-resistant strains had been identified, and the scientific literature on the subject – normally restrained, habitually couched in elaborate conditional clauses – was, for once, plain-talking. The resurgence of plague, and the emergence of new-variant bacilli, were of 'great concern': the reports should be taken as 'warning' of the lurking danger.

In the capital Antananarivo, there were other alarming signs: rats, notably those that foraged in the market gutters and sewers, were developing high levels of resistance to the plague bacillus: trapping was offering up rodents with blood that was aswarm with the infective bacterium, yet the animals were managing to remain unaffected, and lead vigorous, healthy lives. All that was needed for epidemic to strike was a substantial ratfall: in a congested metropolis, rat fleas, their oesophagi engorged with plague blood, would not have to look far for their next hosts.

In an attempt to understand a little more, the Antananarivo branch of the Paris-based Pasteur Institute – Madagascar's biggest disease-research foundation – had started this investigation in two villages high in the central plateaux. Today had brought a whole raft of personnel to one hamlet, the 'test' site: Dr Philippe Mauclère, institute director; head of plague research Dr Suzanne Chanteau; epidemiologist Dr René Migliani; the rat trappers and field workers in their blue overalls; and some sixty or more curious children. Here, for three consecutive nights each month, poisoned bait boxes were set inside houses. Similar boxes were placed in the other village, but these contained unpoisoned placebo bait and plain white flour instead of insecticide powder.

The design of the boxes was cunning yet simple: rectangular, length about four times each end, the interior, when the lid was lifted, revealed three sections of equal size. The two outer contained white insecticide powder or flour; the middle was wedged with three blocks of bait, the size and appearance of Turkish Delight. With the lid down, the ends remained open and beckoning. By enticing rats in, the idea was to monitor numbers by counting their tracks, and then assess the degree of flea infestation and the proportion of both fleas and rats that was plague-infected. The placing of the insecticide either side of the bait – before the rat took its first taste of poison – was crucial: for the experiment not to trigger its own epidemic, the fleas had to be dead before the rat hit the dirt.

Jocelyn Ratovonjato, a young Malgache entomologist with pressed black jeans and a sheaf of laminated graphs, presented his findings. Most compelling were the rat numbers: in the six months of the trial, the totals caught were down by a factor of six, a result that paid testimony to the rat's legendary caution. The rat-track records were yet more telling, clearly demonstrating that, while visits to the poisoned-bait boxes had tailed off, those to the placebo boxes had accelerated. Suzanne Chanteau was smiling.

'They're clever,' she said. 'They've worked it out. It's a bit early to say, but that's my guess.' She paused. 'Rats know when they're threatened. There are records of them sending out their feeblest, oldest members to investigate something they're not sure of. If the old ones die, then the other rats know to stay clear.'

*

SUZANNE CHANTEAU had set the background a few days earlier. She'd driven her Jeep through the crumbling, traffic-snarled streets of Antananarivo to a café to talk. '*La circulation,*' she'd sighed, as the *taxi-brousse* in front of us refused to start, and a group of men climbed out to push it to the kerb, '*c'est infernale.*' In the café, Parisian down to its marble-topped table and white-aproned waiters, she'd drawn an arresting, salutary picture.

To understand why plague had returned so ferociously, she said, an understanding of twentieth-century politics was necessary. Colonized by the French in 1896, Madagascar regained independence in 1960. For a decade afterwards, French institutions stayed largely unaffected. The 1970s, however, heralded military government; Madagascar's own brand of isolationist socialism, 'Christian-Marxism'; and a steady disintegration of the infrastructure – roads, railways, schools, hospitals – of which the French had been so proud. By the 1990s, new democratic government notwithstanding, illiteracy was hovering around fifty per cent and disease was on the rise.

Plague had first reached Antananarivo, in the highlands, in 1921, a long – and still unexplained – twenty-three years after the disease first struck the island. 'Between that date and 1930,' Chanteau said, shaking her head, 'it killed many thousands, but then, in 1931, the first effective plague vaccine came in. There were mass vaccinations. Ten million doses were injected between 1936 and 1960.'

There was a theme here, and it ran pretty much one way: the decline of plague was a colonial success, a triumph of white man's medicine. From 1950, streptomycin and the noxious pesticide DDT were introduced and, over the next thirty years, less than fifty cases a year were reported.

To the alert medic, it must have been clear from the late 1960s that things were going to change. 'The programme for rat-proofing stopped, the old French institutions were left to crumble. The people got poorer and poorer, dirtier and dirtier. Then, in 1978, plague resurfaced in Antananarivo for the first time in almost three decades.'

The rat of choice in Antananarivo – as in any big city – was *Rattus norvegicus*, originally from northern China and southeast Siberia. Unlike the smaller *Rattus rattus*, which preferred houses and, in Madagascar, kept mainly to the red-mud villages in the highlands, *R. norvegicus* revelled in the basest, most derelict areas of urban squalor. In the Analakely district of Antananarivo, there were vast covered markets. In one, smoky soup-and-stew stalls and meat vendors' pitches lined an aisle; behind the haunches of fat-blotched purple beef was a line of cubicles, some shut, most open. Come nightfall, the vendors would bed down here, curled into a corner with their tins and plastic bags and unsold meat. In the gangway running between the stalls, blood and ooze lay in the cracks and fissures, dripping slowly into splits in the concrete that might have been expressly designed for rats. At the far end, in the darkness, was the market toilet: an open door, loose on its hinges, gave onto a heap of excrement and fruit husks, empty tins and nameless mould-encrusted objects; climbing up there, assuming one ever got that desperate, would have involved an all-fours scramble, hands and knees sinking into the mulch and movement of warm decay.

The rats that cruised these districts were showing signs of disconcerting fortitude. Across Antananarivo, Chanteau explained, up to ninety per cent of all rats trapped and autopsied carried antibodies to the plague bacillus: they had, in other words, developed an inherited immunity to plague, born of so many years' exposure.

Chanteau laughed, making light of it. 'Luckily for us.'

Yet it was a delicate balance. To live surrounded by millions of plague-infected rats was sustainable provided the rodents remained alive. If, however, another contagion or an ill-managed poisoning programme caused them to be struck down en masse, then an epidemic of human plague was sure to follow.

The only option, Chanteau maintained, was to aim for a complete eradication of rat fleas with insecticide. 'Unless we do that,' she said, her smile gone, 'we will never stop infection.'

'Could that ever happen?'

'Plague was wiped out in the capital between 1950 and 1978. It can be done.'

In the meantime, the Pasteur Institute and the government health department had joined forces in the struggle against plague. The institute, with its background in research, was stressing the need for 'constant surveillance'. Doctors in the highest-risk plague areas were now under orders to take pus samples from the plague swellings of every single suspected case and send them to the institute, where they were tested for the presence and antibiotic-resistance of the plague bacillus. However, the initial taking of such samples demanded a degree of delicacy that not all field medics – short on equipment and training – possessed.

Often, she said, doctors were helped least by those who should have been most eager to assist: the villagers and slum-dwellers themselves. On some occasions, this was unwitting: because of increasing theft, families had begun storing grain in their bedrooms, thus tempting rats into close contact with warm, sleeping bodies. At other times, as a village doctor would later explain, it was deliberate. Entering areas he suspected to be plague-infected, he'd ask the people if any dead rats had been sighted. For a long time, this line of questioning got him nowhere. Then it dawned: he was asking the wrong question, to the wrong individuals. So he tried the children. 'Can you show me where you've hidden the dead rats?' he'd open, and they'd nod and lead him straight there, to darkened store rooms where there lay in heaps corpses of already balding rodents, orifices gaping and maggot-filled, their fleas – the propagators of plague – long-gone.

In large part, this deception was triggered by fear: that the village would be targeted, that whatever human corpses there were or might be would be seized and impounded and made the target for mysterious, and certainly suspect and undignified, experiments. Few outcomes were more to be avoided, since in Malagasy culture the body of a dead relative was not an empty, worthless husk, but an object of veneration. The magnificent whitewashed tombs in which people from the Hauts Plateaux interred their dead – and from which, at regular intervals, they exhumed the remains, rewrapping the broken skeletons in fresh wild-silk shrouds – were testament to the reverence in which ancestors were held.

This held as strongly today as it had some eighty years before, when the French first launched their anti-plague campaign. As early as 1920, the same deceptive techniques were used to confound the plague inspectors, the French being held guilty of far more than cultural insensitivity: plague, it was claimed, was an invention of the colonizing class, the best way of maintaining ascendancy – germ warfare in its most pernicious and cynical manifestation. This claim gathered momentum until by 1936 – a year of unprecedented revolutionary manoeuvrings – the French administration was being accused by nationalist leaders of unleashing '*une peste politique et raciste*'.

*

MIDDAY, IN A HIGHLANDS VILLAGE some hundred kilo-metres south of Antananarivo. A small crowd stood in front of an abandoned house, home to a traditional healer and part-time astrologer who, some three years earlier, had died of plague. His wife, brother and son had died the same way too, and now the house stood empty, a large spider negotiating the cobwebs that drooped from the first-floor balcony. The door stood ajar, bottom hinge gone. It was dark inside, even though the sun was high, and it was just possible to make out the corner of a table, a plate with something on it.

The healer had been a respected member of the com-munity – second in status, perhaps, only to the village *président* – and his methods of treatment given far more credence than those of the district doctor, with his obscure-

sounding boxes of white pills and predilection for hospitaliz-
ation, evacuation, isolation. So it would have been only
natural for the woodcutter, returning to his home village,
feverish and coughing after a long spell working in a distant
district, to head first for the house of the healer. On the
evening of 20 October 1997, after an arduous day's walk to
Ankafotra, he knocked on the heavy wooden front door. All
that day he'd been hacking up blood, and when the healer
finally appeared, the woodcutter weakly listed his other
symptoms, in particular the pain in his chest, as if someone
had taken an axe to his heart.

He must have badly wanted to get home, must have
had absolute faith in this man, above all others, to cure
him, since he'd endured an extremely tough journey to
reach the village. He'd started out some hundred and fifty
kilometres north, and would have taken endless *taxis-brousse*,
each one more crowded and chicken-heavy than the last,
until finally the track became too fractured and deep-
grooved for even the most determined bush hand to
negotiate with a vehicle.

The healer greeted him and took him inside. Not
realizing that the woodcutter was in the late stages of pneumonic plague – considerably rarer than the bubonic variant
– he opted for his customary blanket approach. Like a
medieval quack, he made a small incision in the woodcutter's chest and sucked out blood, no doubt pausing only to
pronounce a healthy prognosis for his by now severely
delirious patient. Early the next morning, the woodcutter
died.

The healer would have done better to have kept a
good distance. Two days later he was showing identical
symptoms, and three days after that he too was dead. Six

others – three from his own family – would be struck down before the week was out.

One man acted as narrator. He'd been digging a trench with some others and had red mud splattered like blood up his calves and forearms. He'd been a friend of the healer, he said, and had tended him when he fell ill. For six days, he'd sat at the healer's bedside. He wasn't worried about catching the disease.

'I didn't know what it was,' he said. He paused, looking around as if for reassurance. 'And he was my friend.'

After the deaths, the district doctor came back. He warned the villagers of the dangers of rats, how bubonic plague can swiftly turn pneumonic, of the latter's sheer contagiousness. He instructed them, too, in the importance of hygiene, but here, as everywhere else, the houses might have been designed in direct contravention of all the most basic rules of sanitation, specifically with rats in mind: on the ground floor was a dung-trodden enclosure for the family zebu; on the first floor – up, in the gloom, an almost invisible mud-brick staircase – were the kitchen and bedroom and granary, no partitions, mats on the floor. Outside, the earth was swept and there were purple flowers in beds; inside, it was dusty and penumbrous with smoke; touching the walls left fingers smeared black. Despite the petitions of the doctor, nothing had changed.

And what of the healer? Was there a new one, a replacement? Where did the villagers go now for treatment?

Silence. They looked one to another. Then the healer's friend took a step forward.

'The woodcutter,' he said. 'He wasn't from here, you know. He came from somewhere else, some place far away.'

This was untrue: a Pasteur Institute researcher had

documented the case a few months before and, after extensive interviews, had labelled Ankafotra, this village, as 'native' to the woodcutter.

The healer's friend looked at the ground, scuffed his foot in the dust. Across the valley a cock crowed. He looked up again. 'We'd never seen him before,' he insisted. 'He was a stranger to us.'

*

THESE WERE THE STATISTICS: in the fifteen years before 1996, close to twenty-four thousand plague cases were reported to the World Health Organization by twenty-four countries; of these, just over two thousand had been fatal. The worst-affected countries were Madagascar, Tanzania, Vietnam and Peru. Since the early 1990s, the rate of infection had been steadily increasing, which had led the WHO, in 1996, to reclassify plague. No longer dormant, it was now a 're-emerging disease'. Worse, the figures were likely to be wild under-estimates. A 1998 report in the journal *Emerging Infectious Diseases* blamed 'under-reporting in remote areas' and 'the lack of sensitivity of the bacteriological techniques used for diagnosis'.

In the white-neon laboratories of the Pasteur Institute in Antananarivo, Chanteau was working on a small cardboard strip that, she hoped, might change all this. Like an over-the-counter pregnancy test, the prototype was marked, halfway up, with a pink line. Until use, it was stored in an airtight plastic bag. When a doctor took a sample from a plague suspect, all he had to do was inject the pus – or, in the case of pneumonic plague, the blood-flecked sputum – into the bottom of a test tube. Fifteen minutes later, as the strip soaked up the sample, the result became clear: no change meant the patient was free of plague; a second pink line, however faint, spelled infection. A pilot scheme was currently in operation: twenty-five outposts in remote areas, all under orders to test and report every suspect case, to send the finished tests to the institute, treat infected villages with insecticide to kill the rat fleas and, on top of that, 'educate' the inhabitants.

Until now, Chanteau said, plague had been such a problematic disease to diagnose correctly that doctors 'have often preferred to wait and see what happens to the patient. If it is plague, then all that time the fleas are continuing to bite and people are dying.' With a quick-result diagnostic test, she hoped, such fence-sitting would not be necessary.

Yet she was quick to stress her sympathy for the doctors in the field. 'It is not their fault. They have a very hard job. One doctor will have a fifty-kilometre area to cover: that's a hundred villages. He'll have no motorbike, often not even a cycle. *C'est impossible.*'

*

'Dr Chanteau!' The laboratory again. One of her assistants handed over a sheet of paper. It was a printed questionnaire, ruled and boxed. Across the top was printed, '*Fiche Officielle de Declaration Individuelle des Cas de Peste*'. Chanteau scanned it in silence.

At a white-topped table in the middle of the adjoining room sat a man. There was dust in his hair. His collar was so frayed the cotton had split apart. He stared into space as if noticing nothing – the assistants quizzing him in Malgache, the walls covered in charts and pictures of rats and photographs of infected children, Suzanne Chanteau, who moved closer now, beginning her own questioning.

'*Trois morts*,' she said, eventually. 'Three deaths. What happened?'

The man started speaking, his voice a quavering monotone. The assistants translated into French. He'd left early that morning, carrying – on the orders of the district doctor – a test tube with a tissue sample from one of the deceased. He nodded morosely, as if recalling the fifty kilometres of broken roads, the hours waiting in the sunshine for rides that never came, the bewildering commotion and aggression of Antananarivo, his first time in the city.

Two weeks ago, he said, one of the neighbouring children, a three-year-old boy, had fallen sick. The villagers sent for the doctor, but he was not there, and no one knew where he had gone. The child died, but not before infecting his brother. Their father, tending to them, holding the boys as they muttered feverishly, watched them die and then fell sick himself. Four days after burying his children, he too was dead.

'Why,' asked Chanteau – genuinely moved, yet unable to hide her exasperation – 'why did you not find another doctor? *Il faut vite vite voir le médecin.*'

The man did not respond. Chanteau bent closer. 'If anyone has a cough – or anything out of the ordinary – they *must* go to the doctor.' The man, looking down, nodded.

Chanteau looked again at the form. It had been filled in by the stand-in medic, and detailed the symptoms of all three victims. The children were both listed as suffering from classic bubonic plague – engorged lymph nodes, fever, soaring temperatures. The father, however, was not recorded as having had any abnormal swellings.

'Pneumonic plague,' Chanteau muttered to herself. By now, it could have spread further; in the hours it had taken the neighbour to reach the Pasteur Institute, most of the village might have become infected.

Chanteau was shaking her head. She pointed to the form. 'Why weren't they given any medicine – the father, anyone who'd been in contact with the boys?' All the signs pointed to plague – symptoms, speed of contagion – so why wasn't it picked up?

The man shuffled off his stool, got to his feet. He brushed his hands down the front of his shirt. 'We didn't have medicine,' he said. 'And the doctor said it was malaria. We didn't know.' And he turned – his pockets empty, his message delivered – to begin the long journey home.

Chapter Seventeen

AT THE END OF JULY 1894, Alexandre Yersin travelled to
Canton. In Hong Kong, where the hosedown of Taipingshan and the flight of most of its population had seen a
steady drop-off in the rate of infection, he'd assembled
a substantial body of data, taking soil samples from enough
plague-infected houses to offer a reliable ration. 'Four times
out of ten,' he reported, 'I found the microbe.' In houses
where no plague cases had been recorded, the soil was
clean. He travelled to the Chinese mainland to broaden his
research, carrying out the same experiment, with similar
results: the earth in plague houses carried the bacillus 'as
far as twenty, thirty centimetres'. But the presence of the
bacterium did not mean that the soil was necessarily
the source of infection. His next step as good as dispatched the contagious-earth theory so beloved not only of
Kitasato and the Chinese, but also the European medical
establishment: injected with a solution of the bacillus cul-
tured from the soil, not one of his laboratory animals died.
Clearly, another mechanism was at work.

The journey to Canton also confirmed the importance
of what, until now, had been a brief jotting in his notebook:
the epidemic on the Chinese mainland, as he explained
in his 4 August letter to the Governor-General, 'started
with rats; this fact appears indisputable'. There is a surging

detective thrill at this point in the letter, with Yersin under-
scoring 'rat' so forcefully that the pen-mark is still visible
today on the reverse of the page. From his interviews with
doctors, he learnt more: that through February and March
– well before the first human succumbed to plague – 'rats
died in large numbers . . . then the disease extended itself
to men . . . The floating population – very considerable in
Canton – has been almost completely spared.' This was
Yersin at his meticulous, observant best, noting – though
he was still too close to the ground to see the whole landscape, to discern the whole relationship between the
disparate elements of his investigation – the key that would
eventually unlock the mystery of the spread of plague.
The boat-dwellers, he guessed, had been 'spared' because
their homes were inaccessible to rats. As yet, it was only
hypothesis, but he was almost there.

   Back in Hong Kong, Yersin found his contempt deepening for the island colony's management of the plague
crisis. In Canton, not only had he been 'admirably wel-
comed' by the Chinese doctors – in contrast to the continual
rebuff and obstruction he'd received from Lowson – but the
layout of their hospitals and medical treatment was also
markedly superior. The main plague hospital – like his own
hastily constructed *paillotte* – was built from straw. Yet,
despite its emergency construction, considerable thought
had been exercised in the design: each of the twelve hundred patients was accommodated in a separate, clean and
spacious room. By contrast, the Hong Kong hospitals were
notable for their cramped and under-equipped wards: in
Canton, moreover, doctors 'claim to have saved fifty per
cent of the patients'. Mortality in Hong Kong was running
closer to ninety per cent.

To add to his exasperation, he arrived back on the island only to find a letter from Sir William Robinson. Inside, Yersin noted tersely, was a brief note 'demanding again, in my opinion, what would be the measures to take to prevent the return of the epidemic'. His impatience was understandable, for it had been in an attempt to answer this very question – at the first time of asking – that he'd initially begun his soil analyses and then travelled to Canton.

The Governor's previous request for Yersin to investigate the soil inside infected houses had been little more than a cursory duplicate of the instructions issued to Kitasato. Now, however, there was an urgency in his communication. While Yersin was in Canton, Kitasato – after one last tiffin with the loyal Lowson – had weighed anchor and set sail for Japan. He'd packed up his microscopes and surgical instruments, his rack upon rack of tailored suits and dress shoes, and – anticipating a true tickertape welcome, secure in the knowledge that there would be few in Japan still ignorant of his momentous discovery, or of his success against resolute competition – had ordered his research team to board their homeward vessel. He'd left on Friday 20 July – the exact date recorded in large script in Lowson's diary – with the controversy over the discovery still running in the pages of the *Lancet*, and leaving Robinson with no choice but to petition Yersin for help. The Frenchman was now the only choice for a Governor who, with one eye on the approval of his superiors in London, would have realized this one simple fact about disaster management: activity in whatever form is always preferable, and more easily justified, than doing nothing. By attempting to hurry Yersin into the field again, Robinson was covering his back: with his bulletins to the Frenchman diligently copied to Lord Ripon in Whitehall, no one would have been able to accuse him of sitting idly back while the colony slid into oblivion.

It is also possible that Robinson imagined Yersin would have been flattered by the attention: until now, after all, the authorities had treated him with disdain. In his note, Robinson had asked Yersin to stay on for 'a few months more'; only the assumption of a warm reaction could have prompted the Governor to make so large a request. According to Yersin, the colony now wanted him to remain in Hong Kong 'in order to research a practical procedure for disinfecting the soil and to try and prevent a resurgence of the epidemic'. However, his thoughts were already moving on: with news beginning to break about the incursion of plague deep into the Chinese mainland, he knew that containment of the disease within the Far East was becoming increasingly unlikely. A far more radical solution was called for, one that went way beyond the myopic hygiene measures advocated by the Hong Kong government. The answer, he felt sure, lay in effective prevention, and some two weeks after Kitasato's departure Yersin sailed from Hong Kong harbour, bound for Vietnam, where he planned to take the fight against plague on to a whole new plane. With plague now entering new territory, and the causal bacillus identified, he could risk no more time spent in research: action was required and vaccination, he was convinced, was the answer.

He departed as he arrived: alone. To the Hong Kong medical establishment this was the departure of the nearly man, an individual who had – despite Robinson's political insistence on his continued presence – become in the end a figure to be pitied, whose trip to Hong Kong had been one long catalogue of misadventure and missed opportunity. To Yersin's admirers – a mere handful who would, over the years to come, swell to a clamorous multitude – his over-looking remained a mystery that would take another eighty-one years, some three decades after the great man's death, to be conclusively and finally unravelled.

*

KITASATO, ARRIVING IN TOKYO to a slew of adulatory newspaper profiles, launched straight into a series of lectures. The text of these – still available only in Japanese – reveals a confidence and a swagger that speak of a man buoyed up by the adulation of others, at the peak of his powers and popularity.

Seen through the prism of his own words, Kitasato comes across as neither generous-spirited nor open-minded; at home, among peers of his own nationality, he gave free expression to his dislike of European medics in general, while at the same time stressing the bravery and clearsightedness of his own team of researchers.

Particularly dangerous, he explained, had been the post-mortem procedure. The necessary deception and secrecy was 'our greatest difficulty': the moment a patient died, the corpse was nailed into a coffin and 'pretended to be carried to the mortuary in front of the Chinese . . . But actually, the coffin was carried to a hospital room in the police station [now plague hospital].' He continued to outline in minute detail the additional complications. 'We placed the dead body on the cover of the coffin. It was a very uneven floor. This,' he said, indicating the hefty lectern from which he was reading, 'would shake if we placed it on that floor. The room had one window and one entrance. Since

Chinese labourers would walk under the window, we had to close it even when it was hot . . . Yes, the post-mortem examinations were the hardest part.'

Kitasato swelled to fill the role expected of him: returning conqueror, dismissive of the sceptics, secure in his primacy. 'Some people,' he instructed his audiences, 'seemed to doubt my report that I had found the cause of the disease only one week or so after my arrival in Hong Kong . . . I would not express my view irresponsibly, since I am responsible for my field of specialism.'

To his audiences, as in his *Lancet* articles, he gave details of his experiments and the processes by which he arrived at his swift 'discovery'. His 'main goal' in Hong Kong, he explained, 'was to carry out blood tests'. And it was in the blood that he found small quantities of the bacillus; in the spleen and buboes, a far greater volume was present. Having conducted some fifty autopsies, he was convinced. 'I would like to declare, from a bacteriological point of view, that they cause bubonic plague without any doubt.' His bacillus was clearly different from that isolated by Yersin: where Yersin's was larger, more sluggish and did not change colour when stained with alkaline dye, Kitasato's was much smaller and did react to the stain.

His claim staked, he moved quickly to demolish those 'European scholars [who] have mistakenly assumed that plague has vanished from the world'. Such a position, he maintained, could only have come about through severe cultural myopia. Simply because plague had 'ceased to exist in Europe' did not mean that the rest of the world could be regarded as similarly disease-free. 'European scholars should not have made such a conclusion,' he admonished. 'The world consists not only of Europe, but also Asia . . .'

The English medics – who had offered him such whole-hearted support – came in for a forceful drubbing. The slowness of their initial diagnosis struck Kitasato as pre-posterous. 'Even though many Chinese were dying from the plague after it reached Hong Kong, English doctors were not aware of it. This resulted in a rapid increase in the death rate of the Chinese in the spring.' When they 'finally realized' that an epidemic was afoot, 'they found that the symptoms of the patients were very similar to those of the bubonic plague' that are mentioned in old medical books. This astonished the English doctors, and then they went to Canton to trace back to the source of it. However, they faced great difficulties as the Chinese in Canton refused to be examined by foreign doctors and sometimes attacked them. They just beat a hasty retreat to Hong Kong, where the epidemic was raging and the situation was disastrous.'

Kitasato then set about demystifying what he saw as the last veiled area of plague research: the process of contagion. Here too he entertained no doubts: the plague bacillus penetrated the body through a variety of routes: skin, lungs, stomach. His observations of the work of the British soldiers, some of whom contracted plague, had convinced him that the disease 'must have entered into their bodies through the respiration of heavy dust'. Cuts and abrasions were also a risk, he asserted: 'The bacillus may enter . . . through an external wound, which has also been proved by many examples.' What this proof consisted of he did not pause to explain, only adding that 'plague can [also] infect human beings through food and drink'.

Then he took his bow, hearing all around him the applause of his peers, the entire proud nation. There would, he knew, be yet more interviews, more newspaper profiles, quite likely honours from overseas medical institutions, all grateful for his bold pioneering work. He was also expecting a visit from Lowson and – despite his cursory public acknowledgement to the Hong Kong doctor – was planning a lavish welcome, possibly even an audience with the Emperor.

The very last thing he imagined, in this stellar moment, was that the coming decades would witness a gradual chipping away at his reputation and that the worst of the damage, the final work of devastation, would come from one of his own, a respected Japanese bacteriologist with whom, of all people, he would have expected his reputation to be safe.

Chapter Eighteen

IT WAS FIVE IN THE AFTERNOON; dusk was approaching. Yersin, two years after leaving Hong Kong to work in his Vietnam laboratory on the plague vaccine, had been summoned back to the island. Arriving in June 1896, he discovered that the state of emergency had already passed; in Canton, however, plague was running rampant. As the sun dipped over the smoky streets of the city, he found himself filling a syringe with plague serum, about to test it for the first time on a human being.

The patient was a young man, prostrate in the sanatorium of the French mission, with no inkling of what was to come. 'At three o'clock in the afternoon [of 26 June 1896],' recalled Bishop Chausse, the pastor in charge of the mission, in a long letter to the *Hong Kong Daily Press*, 'Dr Yersin came to see me, as he had in 1894.' They shook hands, and the Bishop came straight to the point. 'I said, "Doctor, you have arrived most opportunely. A case of plague has occurred this morning in our establishment, and if you have discovered any remedy for this terrible disease since your last visit, I will be very grateful if you will employ it upon this young man. This case is very pressing, a painful bubo has formed on the thigh, the fever is intense, and the young man is completely prostrated; it is an affair of twenty-four hours." '

Of all the months of preparation, the long days spent in Émile Roux's laboratory in the Pasteur Institute the year before till he was too wall-eyed with exhaustion to look at another slide or culture dish, this was the moment for which Yersin had been waiting and hoping. The vaccine had been tested on animals, but he had no proof that it would be sufficiently powerful to fight plague in humans. From his case he lifted a test tube of the serum – 'a limpid fluid, slightly reddish in colour' – and injected 'a teaspoonful . . . in the skin over one of the hips'. Then he waited.

Darkness fell. Yersin and the missionary sat together a while. Yersin – with an uncharacteristic candour that says much about his fondness and trust for the pastor – 'proceeded to explain the theory of his action by saying that he was going to destroy the microbes by feeding them so to speak, on their own venom'. Chausse, for his part, 'was excited as if going into battle'.

Yersin waited all night at his patient's bedside. At dawn, confident finally that the worst was past, he went to bed. An hour later, Chausse returned to find the patient no longer delirious, but looking up 'with large eyes'. He leant close, and asked how the man felt. The next moments – choked with biblical resonance – gave him a profound thrill. 'The patient replied, "I am cured; the bubo is no longer painful; my head no longer aches." ' Chausse told him, 'Get up and show me that you are cured.' The man sat up, shuffled on his shoes and walked unsteadily about the room. It must have seemed a miracle, an unheard-of reversal of fortune, the kind of transformative recovery that only happened in the Gospels; and, when Yersin came back at nine o'clock, Chausse was puppyish with excitement. 'It is a complete success,' he enthused. 'Your remedy is marvellous;

a thousand times thanks.' Yersin, the true gentleman-
pioneer, deflected the praise. 'It is I,' he answered, 'who
have to thank you, for without you perhaps I should not have
found an occasion to use it.'

*

YET YERSIN, whatever his talent, was alone: one man
against newly resurgent bubonic plague. A hundred years
after Edward Jenner's landmark smallpox vaccination, he
may have become the first scientist to cure a plague sufferer,
but time and numbers were not on his side. By September,
plague had leapt to India, and the Bombay government
was pleading for his help. Whatever the injustices of Kitasato's fame as plague pioneer, the success of the first twenty
or so vaccinations that Yersin had carried out in China was
now well known, and Bombay's request was unequivocal: to
bring as much anti-plague serum to India as he could carry.

*

BOMBAY'S LINK WITH Hong Kong was clear: both were
ports, between which ran frequent commercial traffic. As
one government doctor wrote, '[Since] the outbreak com-
menced near the Docks, it appears most probable that the
infection was introduced by sea and carried in their clothes
or goods by traders who were themselves unsusceptible.'
Like the authorities in Hong Kong, the Bombay government
indulged initially in some energetic wishful thinking: despite
doctors' reports of sporadic cases of patients with suspiciously enlarged glands as early as May 1896, and though
these flared into an unmistakable and full-blown epidemic
in September, it took a further month before the health
department finally acknowledged that the city was experien-

cing an outbreak of 'true bubonic plague'. There was no need, however, for alarm: this was the disease in its 'mild' form.

As in Surat a century later, little heed was paid to the voices of reassurance: between the early-October confirmation of plague until the end of February 1897, an estimated three hundred and eighty thousand people, close to half the population, fled the city. At the height of the plague exodus, only one-fifth of Bombay's millhands remained at their posts. With plague fast spreading into the interior, the government cast around for help, for anyone who might somehow be able to wrest the epidemic back under control. Only one name presented itself, that of Dr Alexandre Yersin, who since the Hong Kong plague summer of 1894 had devoted himself to one task only. For the past two years he'd been working on a vaccine, in the belief that, against a disease of this potency, mankind needed a ring-fence of protection. Plague, for him, had assumed the status of enemy number one: it had to be crushed.

The early narrative of the Bombay outbreak had much in common with the way events had unfolded in Hong Kong. There was the pervasive suspicion of Europeans, born of the fact that relatively few were struck by plague. There was the use of troops to hunt down plague suspects; the widely held belief that the disease was caused by 'overcrowding, destitution, deficient cubic space, ventilation, and sunlight, and a filthy and generally insanitary condition of person, clothing, habitation, and its surroundings'; the suspicion of Western medics as 'callous and patent mercenaries' and hospitals as places of pollution, contaminated by blood and faeces, inimical to caste, religion and purdah. The physical examination of travellers carried out by the mostly white, male cadre of doctors compounded the atmosphere of distrust: a local paper protested in October 1897 that 'Native feeling' was 'most touchy' on this issue: 'Native ladies will prefer death to the humiliation of having their groins examined by male doctors who are utter strangers to them.' Little surprise, then, that families did their utmost to conceal the disease from the search parties. Corpses were buried clandestinely, or stowed in attics, under furniture, inside specially constructed rooms.

Such an atmosphere, with its multiple sources of unreliable information, stoked by fear and hatred, bred rumours of the wildest and most arcane variety. Plague was part of a sinister evangelical plot, some claimed, evidence of a government bent on 'destroying caste and religious observances, with the ultimate design of forcing Christianity on the natives of India'. Others pointed to 'proof' that the government was in the process of poisoning the people: according to one newspaper report, 'six bags of snakes and other worms have been ground [up] and dissolved in the water-pipe at Cawnpore to bring on plague among consumers'. Inside the scrubbed-white wards of plague hospitals all manner of horrors were said to be perpetrated: workers at the Arthur Road Hospital were quoted in one article as believing there to have been 'something diabolical' about a hospital 'which claimed so many victims': patients, it was said, were bled to death through the soles of their feet. There were even rumours that under every hospital bed was an 'oil mill' to grind the patient into ointment for use on Europeans: the plague inspection sheds at railway stations housed, by logical and paranoid extension, 'big machines' for compressing this valuable medicinal ooze from the bodies of innocent Indians. As for the early, unsuccessful attempts at vaccination, these were held to be ruthless efforts at population control: men lost their virility and women became sterile; anyone inoculated was lucky to survive six months; the needle, others said, was a yard long.

To Yersin, such gossip would have seemed close to sacrilege: inoculation, he was now convinced, was the only sure way to curb the spread of plague, and it was to this end that he'd passed the spring of 1895 in his despised Paris. Yet the weeks spent cloistered away in the laboratory would turn 1895 into as historic a year for plague research as that which had just passed. For it was in the Paris Pasteur Institute that Yersin – working with strains of the bacillus that he'd had the foresight to send from Hong Kong months earlier – first demonstrated that a plague vaccine was the best hope against the disease. As an official publication from the World Health Organisation put it in 1954, 'The modern story of vaccination against plague began in 1895 when Yersin, [and his colleagues] Calmette and Borrel proved that the rabbit could be vaccinated against this infection by the repeated injection of microbes killed by heat.'

*

To the Victorian bureaucrat in Bombay, facing social and economic collapse, the request that Yersin simply stockpile a boat with newly manufactured anti-plague serum – and head without delay to India – must have seemed reasonable enough. However, even for an expert bacteriologist such as Yersin, the manufacture of the serum was fraught with uncertainties: it was a delicate process, hard to calibrate, with a raft of unpredictable factors. Firstly, it was dependent on animals.

Back in Nha-Trang at the end of 1896, the telegrams from Bombay mounting unanswered on his desk, Yersin returned to the laboratory he'd set up the year before. Stabled in the grounds were horses, all of which – following the technique first pioneered by Jenner – were in the process of being injected with increasing doses of the plague bacillus. It was the task of Yersin and his team of assistants to then draw off serum – the bile-yellow fluid that separates from blood – that would, by now, be ripe with plague antitoxins. Yersin worked as swiftly as he could, writing to his mother on 20 January 1897, 'As soon as I arrived we did a test bloodletting on two mares who seemed to me the best immunized. If their serum is good I will do big bloodlettings and go immediately to India.' It was a hazardous process, however: horses frequently died, and the wildly varying quality of the serum samples brought Yersin on occasion close to despair.

A month later, he had collected seven hundred doses: cure, if the strengths were correct, and providing they survived the sea crossing, for an equal number of Bombay patients. From choice, Yersin would have stayed longer at his laboratory, but now decided to capitulate, ground down by pressure from Bombay. The texts of India's telegrams to Yersin do not survive, but some significant leverage must have been applied to persuade the Frenchman – who rarely allowed outside pressure, from however elevated a source, to hurry him or force a change of plan – to leave Vietnam before he was ready. Writing again to his mother on 20 February, he did little to hide his resentment. 'It's not seven hundred, but seven thousand doses that I should have been able to take with me, and then my serum would have been able to have been active and effective.' Reluctantly, and despite his misgivings, he began to pack his equipment for the journey.

Chapter Nineteen

BY THE TIME MOHANLAL reached the village, the sun was dipping below the trees. The colour in the sky was fading, turning aquarelle wash. Mohanlal, on the road for almost two days now, was having difficulty focusing. He rested against a fence post and squinted ahead, down the dirt track towards the scatter of low dwellings that was Hetal's parents' home. When he'd first visited he had been astonished that a girl of Hetal's delicacy and urban ease could have been raised somewhere so basic and backward. He, who'd spent his childhood in Bombay and his teens on Chowpatty Beach, found it hard to believe that anyone intelligent could have been satisfied with so little, but he liked her parents: they would speak with hushed reverence of their son-in-law's 'newspaper job', and though they were poor they were hospitable. Now, though, he approached their village in fear: for their reaction to his arrival, for what might have happened to Hetal and his daughter over the past two days, for the future.

He pushed himself upright and, overhead, the vulture that had tailed him for the last hour lifted heavily from the top branches of a skeletal eucalyptus. In the still evening air he could hear the noise of its wings, and a slow clicking sound that he imagined was its beak, the knock of bone on bone.

The village was silent, and he was having trouble recalling the layout, which house belonged to his parents-in-law. He remembered scarlet flowers, some kind of perimeter fence, but that could have been any one of these houses. All were equally humble: cracked mud walls, corrugated aluminium roofs. There can have been no more than twenty or thirty at most, and he was already halfway through. Twenty yards on a tethered goat marked the far limit of the village: beyond were the same terracotta dust fields through which he'd spent the last hours walking, the same concrete-hard earth into which seed, somehow, had been sown.

Someone coughed. Through the darkened window of the nearest house he could see a still candle flame and he turned, called out. No sound. He walked to the door, knocked against the frame. 'Hello?' In the half-light inside he could see two figures sitting motionless on the floor, watching him. A man spoke. 'Further on.' And Mohanlal, seeing them lift their hands to their mouths, retreated as fast as he could, half tripping over a dog in his scurry to reach the safety of the track.

He wanted to cry, but felt too used up and desiccated for tears. He stood very still and felt the cool of darkness come. Now he could see candle glow in all the windows, but still no one ventured outside their doors. Normally, the newcomer to any village faced questioning, invitations from more than one household. The silence now scared him, though he knew it stemmed from their fear of him: they were cowering, as if from a predator, huddled in their furthest, safest places.

Then an older face appeared at a window. In the shadows he could see white hair, a beckoning arm.

'Son!' a voice called out.

Mohanlal broke into a run. Then he was at the door, his ears rushing. His father-in-law was nodding, smiling. His teeth were betel-red, eroded at the roots, and his skin appeared grey, as if he'd not seen rest, much less sleep, in days. 'Son,' he said again, softer now. 'You've come.'

He ushered him inside and, when Mohanlal had crossed the threshold, took one last glance outside then shut and bolted the door.

His mother-in-law was sitting on the floor in front of an open fire. Mohanlal fell to his knees. 'And Hetal?' he said. He could smell the starchy tang of almost-done rice. She raised her pale eyes to meet his. 'Do not worry,' she said. 'You must not.'

The old man was walking slowly to the far corner of the room. He had a limp, and was lifting one heel, his toes dragging. He reached the store-room door, murmuring to himself, and Mohanlal could see his hand moving in his pocket. He pulled out a key and angled the base of the padlock towards him, then pushed the key home. He opened the door and whispered inside.

Mohanlal found himself on his feet. His mother-in-law was holding up a hand but he pushed past her, over the heat of the fire, and in one stride was at the door to the store room.

He heard a whimper, and knew the noise at once. His father-in-law called for a match, and then there was a phosphorous fizz and the store room loomed before them. Hetal was ahead of him, sitting on a grain sack. Their daughter was lying in her lap, and Hetal's eyes were closed; her hand rested on the baby's forehead. Mohanlal's voice came out a croak.

'Hetal, sweetheart. All right?'

His wife nodded, and slowly she opened her eyes and looked up at him. Her neck was blotchy from crying.

'I thought you would not come.' She put a finger to her temple; her breathing was shallow, quick.

He kneeled beside her and inhaled her scent: of the sun, sweet and warm, undercut by something else, something sharper and less familiar. He touched her arm. 'You just left,' he said. 'What was I to do?'

The match died and the store room fell to black again. He got to his feet, lifting Hetal with him. She felt lighter than he remembered, almost insubstantial, even though she was holding the baby too.

'Why are you here?' he asked. 'Why are you hiding away like this?'

She allowed herself to be led to the door; the light from the fire softened the smear of dirt on her cheek, the signs of crying. In her dark eyes he saw the jagged reflection of the flames.

She rested her head on his chest. 'No one knows I'm here,' she murmured. 'It can't get out.'

He nodded and held her and said nothing. He knew she was wrong, had understood this the moment he'd arrived in the village and there had been no one to greet him. He stretched down to touch the baby, but Hetal held the infant tighter, turning away so he could not reach her.

'What has happened?' he said.

But she did not answer nor even, now, meet his eye. Her father put a hand on Mohanlal's shoulder and guided him towards the fire. 'We will eat,' he said.

The rice was overdone, and the curry too heavily fragranced with cardamom. Halfway through he set down his bowl and put out his hand for the baby again. Hetal's mother whispered something to her daughter and Hetal, eyes down, lifted the baby for him to take.

Laying the child in the crook of his lap he immediately noticed a dark ridge of dried blood just above one eye. He touched it, and she moaned in her sleep. He could feel the ridges and grooves of the hardened scab but pulled his hand away, feeling suddenly unsteady. He wanted to wake her, make her cry out loudly and show him she was undamaged.

'What's this?' He tried to sound sympathetic, but could hear the accusation in his voice.

With no warning, Hetal started to speak. She talked fast, as if defying interruption, and her voice rose as she went on, cracking with the release of tension.

They'd been stoned, she said. Like Mohanlal, she'd ridden the train to Anand, but from there no buses would take them and even though she knew she was more of a target on foot, she'd had no choice but to head on. The first night she'd slept in the open, and then, mid-morning, entering a village and desperate for water, had been set upon by a gang of teenagers. She'd shouted that she was holding a baby, but the boys, ignoring her cries, began hurling stones. She yelled back, frightened and bellicose, but that only seemed to fuel their aggression. She was hit on the arm, between the shoulders, and she started to run. She was almost in open country again when a woman stepped out from behind a house and pelted her with a hail of gravel. It was as if in slow-motion, events suddenly suspended, that she saw the skin split on her baby's forehead, the bone-white cut then the first blister of blood; after that it came fast, rich and dark, warm against the cotton of her sari, and she cried out like an animal, a howl that made the other woman, her aggressor, turn and flee.

She ran until she was out of sight of the village and then, under cover of a small spinney, lay her howling baby on the ground and tended to the wound. She tore a strip of cotton from her sari and bandaged the head and for an hour, eyes closed, she pressed a hand to it, feeling the blood under her fingers begin to grow sticky, and eventually the child slept and she was able to strap her again to her chest and move on.

'I will never go back,' she said quietly. 'Not to Surat.'

'Plague will die down,' Mohanlal said. 'Life will carry on.'

She pushed her plate away, shook her head. 'How many people have died? How many?'

He looked from Hetal to her parents: all were waiting, expectant. 'I don't know,' he answered. 'No one seems to know.'

'They wanted to kill me,' Hetal went on. Her eyes bulbed with tears again. 'Just because I came from Surat.'

'But everything we have is there. Our lives, everything.'

She lifted a sleeve to wipe her eye. 'I can't go back.'

'It's plague,' Mohanlal said, trying to soothe her. 'It's not Aids, or some terrible African virus. There is a cure.'

'Plague,' she repeated. 'How much worse can it get? It is 1994, and our city is struck by plague. Doesn't that tell you something?'

Her parents were nodding in agreement now, murmuring encouragement to their daughter, their only child. Mohanlal knew that, against them, he had no words.

'Mohanlal,' she said after a while. 'Mohanlal, my sweet.

Do you want to live in a place where the doctors run away the moment disease strikes?'

He held up his hands, as if in surrender. Less than a week before his world had seemed certain, knowable, unassailable. Now his wife was saying that she wanted no further part of it.

'I don't—' he began to say, but she interrupted him.

'Ghandiji was right. We are a dirty people. We care for our own families, but we are blind to what happens even just outside our own front doors. We do not care.'

Mohanlal suddenly had a picture of similar struggles occurring at that very moment in villages all over Gujarat, wherever Suratis had fled: wives, husbands, grandparents, all arguing over their futures. He did not yet know that, on the world stage, India itself was being shunned, nor that airlines had ceased flights to Indian cities and that some countries had begun imposing embargoes on imports. All he knew was that he would not be the one to run.

'We cannot stay away,' he told her. 'We must go back. Surat is our home, and if we are not to help make it a better place, then who will?'

She reached out, took back the baby. 'That is not my job. I am a mother, and I will not raise my child there.' There was steel in her voice, and he understood that, for them to remain together, only one course of action remained open to him.

'I am tired,' he said. 'I have never been so tired. Tomorrow, we will talk, and we will decide.' He paused. He had no certainties any more, nothing upon which to rest: he could no longer see the future.

'Yes,' he finished, trying to sound as if he had it all worked out. 'Tomorrow it will all be decided.'

*

THE OUTBREAK OF PLAGUE in Surat remained a subject that left no one neutral, that still provoked the fiercest opinion. There was no aspect to the story that escaped controversy; and from diagnosis to treatment, from the intervention of the United States to the fearful reaction of India's trade partners, no single narrative emerged. If there was any agreement at all, it was that a whole raft of culprits was responsible: the federal government, Surat's crumbling infrastructure, the media, America, modern farming methods, the collapse of plague surveillance.

Once again, even the most extreme theories found sympathetic ears. According to the wilder conspiracists, all evidence pointed to a US germ-warfare experiment – a claim loudly rebutted by Washington. The 'proof', so it was said, was various: the presence in Delhi, even before the start of the epidemic, of a team from Atlanta's world-renowned Center for Disease Control; the 'unusual' aspects to the outbreak, in particular the lack of an immediate preceding ratfall and the fact that fewer than a hundred people died, both factors which raised suspicions that this was a 'plague bacterium mutated in some germ-warfare lab'; the disappearance of vital serum samples from the laboratories of Bombay's Haffkine Institute; and the presence in the Surat bacillus of an extra band of protein, too 'fat' to have been the result of natural genetic selection.

Yet the 'whys', as ever, proved more elusive: as the Calcutta *Business Standard* put it, 'What is beyond the comprehension of Indian scientists is why anyone would

engineer a non-virulent strain if it was meant for intentionally introducing plague . . . Some scientists who think the
Surat outbreak was an experiment believe that the aim
could have been to study how the government, the people
and the scientific community would react in the event of a
real attack.'

If the conspiracy-theorists had fingered the US as the
source of the epidemic, a broader consensus also accused
America – in the words of one newspaper – of 'manipulating
public health matters for political ends'. At the heart of
this charge was the alleged glee with which the US media
had reported the epidemic, typified in headlines such as
'Thousands flee Indian city in deadly plague outbreak', and
'Medical experts fear refugees may spread India plague',
both from the normally circumspect *New York Times*.
America, countered India's commentators, was itself a
reservoir of plague, with a steady increase in the number
of cases during the latter half of the twentieth century. So, to
witness its return in India, ran the argument, was an occasion of some satisfaction to the West: 'The general portrayal
of the USA (and Western Europe) as a superior repository
of rationality and civility in a seemingly chaotic world, and
hence ordained for world leadership, is supported by every
successful embarrassment of the Third World.'

Voices of moderation were rare, uncommon the newspaper commentator who strove for balance. Fewer still were
those who chose to look not abroad but inward: plague,
these brave voices claimed, was no one's fault but India's.
Only one writer pointed out, for instance, that the World
Health Organisation had warned as early as March 1994 –
six months before the Surat epidemic – of a global resurgence of plague. 'The most dangerous form of the disease,'

the WHO counselled, 'is pneumonic plague', and it was this of course – which required no ratfall – that hit Surat.

Faced with a collapsed economy and a populace in flight, it took less than a week for India's top doctors and scientists to begin bickering over the cause of the chaos. In Surat itself, there was unanimity: the disease *was* plague, and the city had acted with all speed and efficiency. In Bombay, infectious-disease researchers at the respected Haffkine Institute were less convinced, and drew darker conclusions for the speed of Surat's self-diagnosis, since for the city to have admitted to anything less would have meant that flight had been unnecessary, and the entire disease-control programme a shameful over-reaction. By December, the health department of the Swiss government – which, like so many other overseas authorities, had nervously analysed the chain of events – announced that the outbreak had been nothing less than an 'epidemic in the media . . . It appears that the 1994 outbreak did not take place.' The WHO, it went on, found no evidence of the plague bacillus in man nor animal during the plague weeks, news of which, 'an attentive reader would have observed . . . disappeared from the press on 5 October 1994, the day of the massacre of the members of the Temple of the Sun [a Swiss religious cult]'.

Consensus seemed impossible. Shortly before the Swiss rebuttal, the Center for Disease Control posited the exact opposite, that the outbreak had indeed been plague. The American research had come as a result of an invitation from the Indian government, bamboozled by two months of contradictory findings – first, from Delhi's National Institute of Communicable Diseases and the Surat Medical College, that the disease was plague; second, from the National Institute of Virology and Pune's B. J. Medical College, that it was no such thing, rather a distinct and unrelated infectious disease called melioidosis, whose symptoms conveniently matched those of plague. The CDC report, the government hoped, would be the end of the controversy, and a spokesman for the health department instructed reporters that those 'certain institutions' which registered a non-plague diagnosis had now been ordered to fall into line and 'publicly deny the [earlier] reports'.

To the ordinary resident of Surat, or the inhabitant of any one of the cities to which terrified Suratis were fleeing, these arguments must have seemed at best arcane, at worst an irresponsible diversion from the main business of fighting a disease that was manifestly among them. From the start – while the scientists sniped at one another – the message to the public had been unswerving and direct. Throughout October, billboards across the neighbouring state of Maharashtra had carried 'an appeal' from Information Minister Sharad Pawar. Under a snapshot that made Pawar look bruise-eyed from lack of sleep, the public was exhorted 'to stand solidly behind the government'. His language was steady, his certainty unshakeable. The disease was 'Plague', and originated in the unnamed 'neighbouring state'. In Maharashtra, by contrast, 'the situation is under control . . . Prophylactic measures are being undertaken on a war footing . . . No room should be given to rumours of any type.' As for refugees, he lied, 'their number is minimal'.

*

BUT THERE WAS STILL no resolution. At the Haffkine Institute in Bombay, the country's first dedicated plague centre, the very mention of September 1994 brought sighs of exasperation, hands clapped percussively to foreheads, from the director and his deputies. Here were men who six years earlier had scorned the increasingly desperate communiqués from Delhi's National Institute of Communicable Diseases to 'use masks, wear knee-high socks and gloves, even while sleeping' and who now openly ridiculed those, like the head of Surat's New Civil Hospital Dr Shailendra Vajpeyee, who persisted in talk of plague.

Like the best-schooled politicians, all senior Haffkine staff toed the same line, using identical terminology to describe the outbreak. To Director Dr Barsu Khadse, as to his deputy Dr Narendra Chanderkar and every other Haffkine scientist, the Surat epidemic was 'so-called plague'. There should have been, growled an unsmiling Khadse – a small man dwarfed by a presidential desk, sunk low into a chair whose back loomed a good eighteen inches above his head – no argument.

'I – am – very – busy,' he said. 'Most – exceedingly – busy.' The telephone rang and he answered it with one hand cupped protectively around the mouthpiece. Finishing his call, he spoke in a low monotone, as if to a dictating machine.

'You should know that the Haffkine Institute has very many departments: chemotherapy, pathology, zoonosis, pharmacology, biochemistry, but it was the bacteriology department that in 1994 played such a crucial role in detecting whether the so-called plague epidemic was really plague or not. And we found out that it was not, that it was biochemically different. It was something similar, but not plague. Definitely not plague.'

*

YET ELSEWHERE IN the institute, despite Khadse's prot-
estations, a very different impression was abroad. Every
day, under a plague-monitoring programme that had been
running for fifty years, around fifteen hundred dead rats
were swept off the back of the health department trucks,
combed for fleas and autopsied for evidence of the bacillus.

In the autopsy room, mid-morning, the smell was
already overripe, of blood and excrement, and the technicians in white coats and masks, slicing open rodents in a
line on a long concrete counter, seemed to have their heads
raised as high as possible, as if in an attempt to evade the
stench. By the door were the most recent deliveries: five full
buckets of rat corpses, their bodies twisted around each
other, mouths yawning open, their clogged and matted fur
the only sign of the drowning that had been the cause of
death.

Every night, from the urban heart of Bombay to its
dishevelled suburbs, teams of rat catchers baited cages,
returning each dawn to catch and drown the rodents and
deliver them to the institute. From each district too, a small
number was always kept alive and here, in the centre of the
autopsy room, was a cylindrical concrete holding tank,
about eight feet across, where the animals were allowed to
run free until fresh blood was required. In the corner of
the room were filmy yellow garbage bags, full of old test
tubes, banana skins, discarded masks, and dismembered
and discarded rats that pushed fatly against the translucence
like an intruder in a fifteen-denier mask.

A technician looked up. 'I hope,' he murmured, 'that
no one still believes that there was any kind of controversy.
Here at Haffkine there is no disagreement. Bombay had no
plague, nor the whole of Maharashtra state.' He was silent

a while, then shook his head as if in stern disapproval.
'There was no plague in Bombay,' he repeated dully. 'This
city, our city, did not have plague.'

*

AN UNSETTLING PICTURE was emerging, one in which a
misplaced kind of regional loyalty had become more
important than truth, however unpalatable. It was as if even
to raise the subject, merely to pose the question, was seen
almost as wilful provocation. Only in the broadest historical
or theoretical discussion, it seemed, was one safe, and later
a technician led the way through the laboratories where
serum was plague-tested, outlining the three tests that
'ensure that no case goes undetected'.

'The first two tests,' he announced eagerly, 'the first two
are staining and microscope analysis. You know what the
bacillus looks like? Like a safety pin, exactly. So we look for
that. Also we see if there is bipolar staining. Finally, just so
we are completely sure, we take serum samples direct from
the hearts of the rodents and test for plague antibodies.'

Through another microscope he showed me a slide of
Xenopsylla cheopis, the rat flea. Under magnification the flea
looked bigger than the lens, suddenly swollen monstrous.
Its legs were most striking: long and muscular and hairy,
multi-jointed.

'That is the real villain,' he said. 'That is why we say
that people should not sleep on the ground during plague.
When rats die, the fleas search for other hosts, but they
cannot fly, so during epidemics people should make their
bed at least one foot above the ground.'

Slowly, out of earshot of the offices of the Haffkine
management, the technician was getting back on to territory

that no longer smacked of news management. Plague, he went on, was a disease that required constant monitoring. The fact that Bombay had not seen 'classical plague' since 1966 meant little.

'It is out there in the forest, in the countryside, all the time. We have different people from the health department killing the rats there, doing surveys. If plague spreads from the countryside to the city it will create havoc. It is,' he said, his jaw set, 'a very dangerous disease which is always just around the corner.'

He was out of the cool of the laboratories now and was standing on the first-floor balcony, overlooking the main sweep of drive where once, when this had been the Governor's residence, elegant landaus would have ferried white-suited civil servants and their soft-voiced consorts to endless cocktail receptions, but where now, a century on, the only sign of human life was a single desultory gardener directing an aimless hose at the poinsettia. The technician had begun to talk more widely about plague, its spread in the modern world.

'No one talks about America, do they?' he burst out. 'They've had outbreaks of plague in the twentieth century. There are reservoirs of plague in the wild rodent population in the western United States, but how much do you read about that? Every year people get plague in America, but does it get reported? A single outbreak in India, and the whole world is cancelling holidays, boycotting our products, and stopping our planes from landing.'

Chapter Twenty

OVER THE CENTURIES that plague had lain quiescent, remaining always an opaque threat, it had acquired the status of some kind of diabolical sorcery. According to one chronicler, it was the 'Flying Dutchman of disease' because of its seemingly magical ability to traverse the earth and explode in areas and at times when it was least expected. In the last two years of the nineteenth century, plague – from the flashpoint of Hong Kong, in 1894 – flared in Arabia, Mauritius, Japan, Algeria, Mozambique, Turkey, Russia, Egypt, Africa, Paraguay, Turkestan, Austria, Brazil and Madagascar. In 1900, it hit Manila, Hawaii and the United States.

Its spread across America – and the resultant lingering threat that it poses even today – remains one of the nation's most effectively buried pieces of medical history. From the first US human plague death in March 1900 in San Francisco, the disease spread steadily until by 1905 – after successive San Francisco epidemics – it broached Oregon and Washington State. In 1906 it struck Louisiana; eight years later New Orleans fell victim; and, by the end of the decade, Florida and Texas were also affected.

Pneumonic plague was not recorded in America until it hit Oakland in 1919. Five years later, in Los Angeles, the pneumonic variant struck with such startling force that the entire county was mobilized in an effort at containment. Once again – and gratifyingly for the vocal white majority who held that disease was something that happened only to the primitive other – plague overlooked the Caucasian districts, and ignited in an area inhabited almost wholly by Mexican immigrants.

First to die was Lucena Samarano, owner of a boarding house at 742 Clara Street. With no epidemic suspected, no inquest was held, but three days later, 22 October, her husband Guadalupe Samarano, and Jessie Flores, a nurse who had cared for Lucena, both fell sick, complaining of high fever, back pains and 'expectorating' – in the words of the California State Board of Health report – 'a profuse bloody sputum'. They died soon after, and in the days that followed, a large number of their neighbourhood was also struck down.

It took a good week for correct diagnosis to come through, and the response of the city – armed now, thanks to the work of Yersin and Paul-Louis Simond, his successor in India, with both understanding and methodology – was immediate and determined. Eight city blocks – comprising most of the Mexican population – were cordoned off and quarantined. Seventy-five police officers patrolled the perimeter; sentries were also posted outside houses where cases had occurred and further infection was predicted. Ration packs were delivered to all houses under quarantine, and the Macy Street Baptist Church was seconded as a laboratory for rat dissection. With quarantine enforced and daily house inspection underway, the focus moved towards rat extermination, since for two decades now rodents had been established as the primary carriers of bubonic plague, from which pneumonic plague then sprang. According to the Health Board, 'Trapping operations were started, the entire local supply of traps was obtained, telegraphic orders sent to San Francisco for all available traps and arrangements [were] made with eastern firms to rush their entire supply to Los Angeles. A total of forty thousand traps was thus obtained.'

It was an all-American operation, carried out with an uncomplicated sense of moral purpose and more than a hint of pious self-congratulation: the weekly meetings of the Health and Sanitation Committees, the numberless sub-committees busying themselves with ever-more civic-minded 'recommendations', the creation of a dedicated Rodent Control Department, the fulsome $750,000 'budgetary appropriation' for fighting plague, all this and more spoke of a state government in reassuring and masterful control. Plague suspects were dispatched to the same hospital, the Los Angeles General, where they, their wards and charts were tagged with prominent red labels. The hospital – an archetypal early-century institutional edifice, its windows vast and square, its slab sides zigzagged with cast-iron fire escapes – issued a daily 'plague bulletin', detailing numbers of deaths.

The Health Board report divides into dark and light, black and white. Nowhere is this more evident than in the selection of photographs. Dark is disease, and the neighbourhood from which it came: it is the 'shack used as sleeping quarters' at the back of 742 Clara Street, shot at sundown, the rough-boarded dwellings in deep brooding shadow; it is the 'typical interior of Mexican home', bed and chairs strewn with clothes, upturned chests serving as kitchen cabinets, bucket as garbage pail filled to overflowing with empty bulk cartons of Camel cigarettes; it is the blurred focus of 'premises, North Anderson street, where two bubonic plague cases occurred', the whole scene redolent of ribbon development along a railroad track, unplanned and unchecked, from which the well-heeled, riding towards open country, would carefully avert their gaze.

Light, through a choice of photographs that was no doubt largely subconscious, is associated with the white man and his righteous endeavours to curb disease. While 'the Mexican', like 'the oriental' in Hong Kong, was seen as a homogeneous racial type, who 'always, when ill, calls the Priest, and generally [is] prompt in securing medical aid', pictures of the American doctors and the gleaming-floored plague wards encouraged an impression of a world where malign forces could hold no sway. The white medics were portrayed as resourceful and innovative: in the absence of ready-made supplies, masks were made from pillowcases, with 'celluloid eye pieces' and 'gown fitting closely about the neck': latter-day Ebola paramedics, every inch of skin concealed. So, with perfect propagandist logic, America's worst outbreak of pneumonic plague – though small in fatalities, accounting for just thirty lives – was transformed, to become a totem of hope for the future.

One image prevails: that of a Mexican boy, six-year-old Raul Samarano, sole survivor of 742 Clara Street and, according to the caption, 'the only child known to have recovered from an attack of pneumonic plague'. What is most striking is not the plain fact of his survival, but rather the photographer's knowing juxtaposition: the startling white bars of his hospital cot against the tan of his face, his tiny form surrounded by the very image of the modern world, the confident, healthful future: a place where plague would find no home.

*

YET IF HISTORY HAS anything to teach us about plague, it is that it refuses to be reined in. If diseases have personalities, plague is an escape artist, a criminal Houdini, tunnelling from the highest-security confinement to trigger new outbreaks, to wreak escalating havoc. Its quiet periods are illusory, time during which – as the antibiotic-resistant strains in Madagascar have shown – it is mutating, regrouping for fresh attack.

After the 1924 Los Angeles outbreak, the disease consolidated its position, digging in as if for a long siege. Through the first half of the twentieth century, few years escaped without plague being reported in America, and as the disease spread eastward, through the Midwestern prairie states towards Florida, Texas and Louisiana – crossing the Sierra Nevada mountains in 1929 and the Continental Divide in Montana four years later, to reach Canada by 1942 – so the numbers of infected animal species multiplied. In 1902, three species of US rat were known to be carrying the plague bacillus; by 1940, the figure was forty. The picture was the same with fleas: in 1900, after the late-nineteenth-century work of Paul-Louis Simond in northwest India had proved the role of flea as plague vector, just five different kinds were under suspicion of being carriers; four decades later, some thirty-five fleas had been associated with the disease.

Today, hikers and hunters out bush in the western states are at risk from a bewildering number of animals: infected mice were found in Louisiana in 1915; ground squirrels in

California in 1908; ground hogs some twenty years later
in Oregon; and prairie dogs, marmots, Tahoe chipmunks
and kangaroo rats have also all tested positive. It is this
ever-present, constantly refilling reservoir of plague that
continues to pose a danger into the twenty-first century:
in New York, a city thus far free of plague, the Health
Department has gone to the trouble of posting a page on
its Web site detailing the symptoms of plague, and the
current best treatment routes. Lessons have clearly been
learnt: with plague, nothing less than constant vigilance,
unflagging surveillance, will do.

*

YERSIN, CARRYING HIS seven hundred doses of pioneering
anti-plague serum, docked at Bombay harbour on 5 March
1897. A scene of eerie calm would have greeted him as the
hills of Bombay emerged from the heat haze: the dock,
normally chaotic with activity, clamorous from the hollering
of fishermen and cargo hands, was now absolutely still: not
a boat moved. Stepping ashore, he'd have quickly discovered
the reason: the imposition of quarantine, intended to
prevent the further spread of plague, had resulted in the
effective closedown of the port, of all international trade.

The atmosphere in the city itself – the simmering
loathing that Europeans and Indians reserved for each other
– would have brought back uncomfortable memories of
Hong Kong. This time, however, Yersin, at least in French
eyes, was no longer the unknown ship's doctor and part-
time jungle explorer who had arrived to such indifference
in Hong Kong harbour that June evening in 1894. Here
was now a man who – if one left aside the ongoing tussle
for the title of true plague pioneer – had proved himself

fully in the field. It was he who'd spent the last two years working on a vaccine, he who quietly assumed that, given time, he would emerge from Kitasato's overblown shadow, and now it was he who was once more risking his life on the frontline.

For the next two months he was the guest of the French Consul, and his days and nights cannot have struck a greater contrast. By day, he sought out the most abandoned and diseased parts of town; by night, he returned to the butlers and polished hallways of the consulate, his foie gras and chilled Chablis awaiting him, the sheets of his bed pressed and freshly scented. Aided this time by the authorities – rather than, as in Hong Kong, wilfully obstructed – he pushed on with his vaccination programme, but the results were disappointing: barely half his patients survived. The arrival from Paris of a batch of Pasteur Institute vaccine – a process initiated by Yersin in France the year before – saw his spirits rise, and something of his old optimism return. With the Paris preparation, closer to eighty per cent recovered.

Yet, as the weeks wore on, a familiar pattern began to emerge. The Bombay government, reacting no doubt in part to Yersin's often blundering negotiating manner, started restricting his access to plague patients: to Yersin's frustration, he was too often only allowed to carry out injections when the patient's infection had become irredeemably advanced. Fury then exhaustion set in and when in July he received orders from the Pasteur Institute to return to his laboratory in Nha-Trang, he did so almost gratefully, with no hint of rivalry in the welcome he gave Dr Paul-Louis Simond, the bacteriologist sent to replace him.

And so 'the intrepid Yersin' – as Louis Pasteur had

dubbed his young disciple – settled back into life in Vietnam, concentrating on establishing a specialist immunization laboratory and heading the small community of cattlehands, technicians and farmers required to keep such an enterprise in operation. In his own mind, he was convinced of the credit that – as the first to isolate the cause of plague and the pioneer of the first anti-plague vaccine – was rightly his, yet must have wondered, as he forged on alone in his fight against the disease, whether he was destined to live out his days unacknowledged and overlooked, in the eyes of the scientific community no more than the dramatic foil for the true hero, Shibasaburo Kitasato.

*

SIMOND, FELLOW PASTEURIAN, was one of the few for whom Yersin's reputation was unassailable, and he arrived in Bombay flattered and thrilled to have been asked to take over the senior bacteriologist's work. What he had not prepared for, however, was the volatile parabola of plague, and his first few weeks in the city in the May of 1897 brought an unexpected – albeit temporary – quiescence. Yet this lull also carried opportunity, and Simond, demonstrating a hunger for the big prize that might have been learnt at Yersin's knee, seized the chance to home in on the one major remaining unknown of plague research: the process of transmission.

Until now, the boldest rat–plague connection had been made by Yersin himself, three years earlier in Hong Kong: '*Il est probable,*' he had written in his notes, '*que les rats constituent le principal véhicule.*' Yet this was hypothesis, and had been taken no further. It was also, to judge from

prevailing opinion in Bombay, a theory that was pitiably
wide of the mark.

On the Indian west coast, all efforts were focused on
disinfection, segregation and quarantine: logical consequences, in the eyes of Bombay medics, of the discovery of
a specific bacillus of plague. Consensus was in favour
of human-to-human transmission, and maximum energy
was being expended in attempting to track down and isolate
infected persons: along all railroads and main arterials
checkpoints were set up, and fugitives searched and medi-
cally examined. The disinfection operation was equally
formidable, with some thirty-one thousand Indians hired
by the government as emergency street, house and sewer
cleaners. Such was the volume of carbolic acid used in the
sluicing of houses that health inspectors would cower under
umbrellas as they entered buildings, as protection from the
corrosive spray from the upper storeys. Every day, three
million gallons of disinfectant were pumped into the sewers;
grain was either burned or laid in the open to 'breathe'. In
the midst of all this poisonous commotion, the rat escaped
the city unnoticed, spreading infection as it went.

Simond, settling in, would have brought himself quickly
up to pace with the latest research and hypotheses of the
international plague missions stationed in the city. In large
part, these were substantial posses of government-sponsored
scientists – from Russia, Germany, Britain, Austria – all of
whom had staked out firm, and for the most part equally
erroneous, claims about the mechanism of the disease.
According to the German Plague Commission, parasitic
insects were manifestly not to blame: if they had been, ran
their argument, the plague hospitals would surely have been
worse hit. The Austrians' blind fumble towards a solution

concluded that any kind of irritable scratching of the skin
might lead to infection. The British, while conceding that
infection normally happened through the skin, rejected the
notion of blood-sucking insects as vectors of plague: usually,
they suggested, soil was the area of highest danger, with
exposed microbes the likely agents of transmission. Rats
were mentioned but briefly, and when they were it was in
a tone of almost flippant dismissal.

Yet the rat – to judge from plague accounts from previous epidemics – clearly merited closer attention. In the
East, the connection had been made as early as the tenth
century: the noted Arabian physician Avicenna, who lived
in Persia between 980 and 1037, had described how the
appearance of plague would cause an unsteady, stumble-
footed exodus of rats and other subterranean animals from
their burrows. In London in 1665, observers noticed a
similar chronology: Nathanael Hodges' *Loimographia*, an
account of the London plague of 1665, gave as 'a sure sign
that pestilence is at hand' the startled and sudden emergence of moles, mice, serpents and foxes from underground.
In China, a century later, the first suspicions of a causal
chain were beginning to emerge: of the Yunnan outbreak
of 1792, Hung Liang-Chi wrote that it was rats that died
first; human deaths came later. The rodents, he added, were
everywhere and unavoidable, appearing as never before in
broad daylight, vomiting blood as they staggered their final
steps.

Simond's first observation was startlingly different to
those of his peers, and indicative of a man unencumbered
by the herd instinct that distinguished the thought process
of most of the international plague commissions. Examining
the symptoms of plague patients in an epidemic hotspot

some way up the coast, he noticed the occasional presence
of a tiny blister on the feet and lower limbs. This in itself
was a fairly workaday observation, and one that had moreover been made by numerous other plague researchers:
where Simond differed was in his level of curiosity. Taking
the trouble as no one had before to examine microscopi-
cally the fluid drawn from the blister, he found a swarming
abundance of plague bacilli. His resulting hypothesis was
the beginning of a theory of plague transmission that would
cause him to suffer ridicule for the rest of his life and for
which he would only posthumously receive credit.

Working under conditions uncannily reminiscent of
those endured by Yersin in Hong Kong – instead of a
grass hut, Simond had just a small tent to protect him, his
experimental instruments and animals from the onslaught
of the Indian monsoon – he demonstrated the kind of
bravery for which Yersin was already well known. As he
learnt more about the likely mechanism of transmission, a
fearful recoil would have been understandable enough, yet
his behaviour betrayed no such trepidation. He would have
known that science conferred no immunity from plague –
one of Kitasato's team had died from an infected scalpel
cut in 1894 – but this did not deflect him. He was closing
in, and would not turn back.

Insects had already been implicated in disease transmission, and Simond would certainly have been conscious
of Patrick Manson's 1877 experiments in China which
showed that the mosquito was a factor in the spread of
systemic filariasis, just as he would, some four years later,
have read of Carlos Finlay's proposal that the causative
agent of yellow fever was also carried by mosquitoes. Yet,
though time would vindicate their theories, such thinkers

were as yet considered near-heretical by the scientific mainstream, with Finlay's work, for instance, earning him the sobriquet of 'theorizing old fool'. For Simond even to consider and begin investigating such a mechanism for plague – so setting himself up in opposition to the accepted wisdom of international science – was courage in itself.

Researching alone, he determined to ignore the encroaching barrage of conflicting hypotheses and concentrate instead on his own observations. Working from no one's notes but his own, he observed and distilled, sifting relevance from red herring. His notes are simple, unadorned: he wrote down only what he could see and what he was told: he was baffled, intrigued, utterly focused.

From the start, it was clear that the most popular theory of contagion – through either air, food, or infected faeces – merited no further respect. Most striking, for Simond, was the almost spectral, random manner in which the disease appeared to surface, often finding new victims at considerable distance from those already infected. He recorded instances of plague flaring up in houses a good half-mile from the next nearest case, whose inhabitants claimed to have had no contact with other plague sufferers. A carrier, Simond posited, was at work, and, like Yersin before him, he fingered the rat.

Drawing on his experience in the field, he recalled that, in China's Yunnan province, people fled their homes on the first sight of a dead rat; in Taiwan, any contact with dead or dying rats, however fleeting, was believed to lead to plague. As he travelled the worst-hit plague districts of Bombay and beyond, evidence was building: his notebook contains a description of one house in Karachi in which no less than seventy-five dead rats were found. Standing in the street, wondering where to position this latest piece of the jigsaw, he witnessed the trademark drunken shambolic stagger of the plague rats, animals uncommonly oblivious, their usual nimbleness gone, dragging their limbs, dying in front of him in the dust.

Yet if rats were to blame, it remained uncertain exactly how the plague bacillus made the leap to humans. At issue, Simond judged, was chronology: some kind of sequence was in operation. A Bombay wool factory offered up a crucial clue, recorded by Simond in his characteristically exact prose: 'One day, employees arriving in the morning noticed a large number of dead rats on the floor. Twenty labourers were ordered to clean the floor of the dead animals. Within three days, ten of them developed plague. None of the other employees became ill.'

Simond had broken from the pack, and from this point on was on his own. Deliberately, now with only half his mind on the vaccination programme, he sought out survivors, juicing them for information. Increasingly, his questions followed a similar track: Did rat mortality precede human deaths? What contact had the deceased had with dead rodents? In some villages, like one he visited in April 1898, the people appeared to intuit the process at work with far greater accuracy than did the theorizing luminaries assembled in Bombay: in this particular village, Simond noted, the population had fled their homes the moment news spread of the first dead-rat sighting. 'Two weeks later, a mother and daughter received permission to go back to the village to bring clothing from their house. They found several dead rats on the floor of the house. They picked up the rats by their tails and threw them out on the street and then returned to the camp. Two days later, both developed

plague.' These are a detective's notes, written hastily, anticipating no further readership: there is a winning modesty,
too, as well as the kind of self-restraint exhibited by Yersin.
Simond, employing the same deadpan prose which he might
have used to murmur confidences to a colleague, listed 'one
more observation: on 13 May 1898, in Bombay, a man
walked into a stable to take care of his horse and found
there a dead rat on the floor. He picked up the rat by the
tail and threw it out. Three days later he developed plague.'

A perplexing picture was beginning to emerge, one in
which a dead rat, contrary to expectations, appeared to be
far more dangerous than one captured alive. There was
clearly a missing link, and Simond already had more than
enough evidence to implicate the rat flea, *Xenopsylla cheopis*.
In the Karachi house, reluctant home to the corpses of
those seventy-five rats, fleas were found darkly swarming,
shadowy swells of movement. 'On the rats captured alive,
and on the rats which had just died, the fleas,' wrote
Simond, 'were thicker than I had ever seen them.' And so,
tentative at first, came the hypothesis: 'We have to assume
that there must be an intermediary between a dead rat and
a human. This intermediary might be the flea.'

Step by step, his research was becoming more and more
perilous, and the next move towards proving his hypothesis
was the most hazardous yet. In order to establish whether
the flea was the go-between, he first had to discover
whether it was capable of absorbing and transporting the
bacillus. In Cutch-Mandvi, a town north of Bombay in
the maw of a ferocious outbreak of plague, and to which
Simond had just been posted, he devised an experiment
that was as fearless as it was direct. Trawling the back alleys
until he found a rat that had died recently enough to be

still blood-warm, he seized it with long forceps, dropped it into a paper bag and rushed the whole parcel back to his tent laboratory. Here he sank the bag into a tub of warm soapy water, scissored it open and combed a scattering of drowned fleas from the matted fur of the rat. Compared to insects taken from a healthy rat, their intestines showing nothing abnormal, fleas from the plague rat were bloated with the bacillus.

The final section of the search for proof – carried out in Karachi, in the spring of 1898 – bears the genius stamp of simplicity. With limited materials and laughably basic clinical surroundings, Simond devised an assay so unpretentious, so Boy-Scout straightforward, that it was inevitable that it should attract ridicule from the regiments of sophisticated science. One can almost picture him arranging on a bench his few tools and experimental objects, explaining the process step by step, as if an easy-smiling presenter on a parentally approved children's television show. He laid out a wide-mouthed glass bottle, some sand, a strip of fine wire mesh and the same length of cotton fabric, a metal cage small enough to fit into the bottle and finally two rats, one obviously ailing, one in bouncing health.

The plague rat Simond 'was fortunate enough [to have caught] in the home of a plague victim. In the rat's fur there were several fleas running around. I took advantage of the generosity of a cat I found stalking the hotel premises, borrowing some fleas from it.' He emptied the sand – a urine-absorber – into the bottle, dropped the rat in on top, and 'deposited the cat's fleas on it from a test tube. I was thus quite sure the rat would be covered with parasites.'

Like a dispassionate seven-year-old frying ants with a magnifying glass, Simond then watched as the rat began its final contortions. Twenty-four hours on, the animal had 'rolled up into a little ball. With its hair standing on end it seemed to be in agony.' Knowing that death was now near, and that the rat's plague-engorged fleas would, as soon as they sensed the rodent's body begin to cool and stiffen underneath them, be looking to move off in search of warmer and fresher blood, Simond then 'introduced into the bottle a small metal cage containing a perfectly healthy young Alexandria rat caught several weeks before and kept sequestered from any danger of infection. The cage was suspended within the inside of the bottle several centimetres above the layer of sand. The cage had three solid sides, but the other three sides were covered by wire screen with a mesh size of about six millimetres. The rat inside the cage could not have any contact with the sick rat, the wall of the bottle or the sand.'

The next morning, the first rat was lying cold on the sand. Simond left it another twenty-four hours, then removed it for autopsy. 'The blood and organs all contained an abundance of [plague] bacilli.'

Again, notepad at his elbow, he sat down to watch. For four days, the caged, healthy rat continued to feed and sleep normally. Then, on 'about the fifth day, it seemed to have difficulty moving. By the evening of the sixth day it was dead. An autopsy of this one revealed buboes, both inguinal and axillary. The kidney and the liver were swollen and congested. There were abundant plague bacilli in the organs and blood.'

From theory to practice, from hypothesis to first proof, Simond's experiment and its robust conclusion was like an adrenaline punch to the heart. His involuntary yelp of realization, in all its unrestrained and maximum-decibel joy, deserves to be printed in full. '*Ce jour-là, le 2 Juin 1898, j'éprouvai une émotion inexprimable à la pensée qui je venais de violer un secret qui angoissait l'humanité depuis l'apparition de la peste dans le monde.'* 'That day,' he fizzed, 'I felt an inexpressible emotion at the thought that I had just uncovered a secret that had tortured man since the appearance of plague on the earth.'

Simond's findings, under the title *La Propagation de la Peste*, were published in the Pasteur Institute journal that same year. His recommendations were as penetrating and unstinting as the accounts of his research. The key to controlling plague, he said, was keeping rat populations in check: port authorities should do everything in their power to prevent rats jumping from ship to shore; any vessel coming from an infected area should be fumigated with sulphuric acid. In these strictures, as in his findings, he was the lone voice, the prophet without honour: not one scientist, from any of the assembled international commissions, held up his work for anything but scorn. Typical was an editorial comment in the *Indian Medical Gazette* some four years later which referred to similar – but crucially flawed – experiments by the distinguished Cambridge parasitologist George H. F. Nuttall as 'having pretty completely demolished Simond's . . . worthless . . . flea hypothesis'.

History has treated Simond little better: he remains a forgotten hero whose name is often conspicuously absent from works of medical history, in which chapters dealing with the race to find the cause of plague refer to those who built on his pioneering work, and seldom to the trailblazer himself. In part this may have been down to Simond's personality: notably uninterested in the egotistical scramble up the ladder of doctorates and professorships, he was described by a pupil as being 'without ambition, indifferent to things he knew only too well to be vain, devoting himself [in old age] to his friends and giving himself over to social work for the betterment of his neighbours'.

Yet he was equally likely to have been overlooked as the deliberate result of professional jealousy. This is more than fancy: in Victor Heiser's bestselling travelogue *An American Doctor's Odyssey: Adventures in Forty-Five Countries*, the peripatetic medic referred to 'a hypothesis conceived by P. L. Simond of Spain [sic] that plague was conferred by fleas. He had no supporting proof for his theory; he merely imagined this was the way it happened. His claim was tested first by the First Indian Plague Commission which, after investigation, announced that no connection could be found between the flea and the rat.' Heiser's information came from a visit to India in 1902, during which he was befriended and escorted around the plague hospitals by one of the most senior members of the Indian Medical Service. No doubt to the sweet satisfaction of his source, he made no attempt to seek any response from either Simond or the Pasteur Institute.

Amazingly, nowhere in any of Simond's papers can one detect a hint of resentment Awarded the Légion d'honneur in Paris in 1901, he went on to study yellow fever in Brazil, found a medical school in Marseilles and serve as Director of the Imperial Institute of Bacteriology in Istanbul. He retired to Valence, in a house on whose walls were skins from a Bengal tiger and leopard: talismans from his travels. He wrote and published short stories, could run off an accomplished piano sonata and was, until old age, a patient and intuitive trout fisherman. He died on 18 March 1947. On his gravestone is carved but a single line: Docteur P.-L. Simond, 1858–1947. No bombast, no plea for immortality. Just a profession, a name, some dates.

Chapter Twenty-One

By 1907, THE WORK BEGUN BY Simond in 1898 – and expanded, consolidated or just plain plagiarized by each wave of successors – had become established scientific fact, as uncontroversial a notion as the orbit of the earth around the sun. For the Citizens' Health Committee of San Francisco, struggling to beat back plague after the earthquake and city fires of that spring, the aim, in the words of committee historian Frank Morton Todd, was simple: 'to organize the community for the starving and destroying of rats'. Yet for this to succeed among a populace wholly ignorant of Simond's rat-flea thesis, some significant re-education was required. The city, Todd explained in his colourful prose, 'had to go to school and study zoology, bacteriology, and fleas. The whole community had to learn about plague as a disease and an epidemic. In general, this is what it learned. Bubonic plague is not a filth disease – it is a rat disease.'

The war on the rat was waged with a specifically military lexicon. Photographs of the 'regiments of health' show ranks of black-suited, trilby'd conscripts, brooms shouldered as if they were .303s. Every day they set up scores of poison-baited traps. The poison – a mixture of 'phosphorus or arsenic baited with lard, cheese, sugar or other food preferred by rats' – was 'spread on stale bread' and placed inside nineteen-inch wire-cage snares, and circulars were rushed out describing in detail how and where the traps should be most effectively set. These instructions were clearly intended for householders not much accustomed to rat destruction – 'Before setting, the lever on the trap should be tested to see that it works properly' – and gave considerable space to the rodent's catholic taste in scraps. 'The rat is more or less of an epicure; therefore the bait should be changed at frequent intervals. Also, he should be given food which he is not in the habit of getting. For example: in a meat market, vegetables are the best bait, while in a location where vegetables are plentiful, fresh liver and fish heads or a little grain are best. The following may be suggested as good bait to be used: fish, fish heads, raw meat, cheese, smoked fish, fresh liver, cooked corn beef, fried bacon, pine nuts, apples, carrots and corn. When trapping in chicken yards a small chick or duckling is remarkably good.'

Dealing with an animal with the boundless cunning of the rat required a degree of sly forethought. Females could even be used as lure to 'call in the young or the males'. Final touches were equally important: 'Before leaving the trap, it should be smoked with a piece of burning newspaper to kill the smell of the human hands or rats which have been in it.' The rat, ran the subtext, was a notable adversary, and exterminators were instructed to be ever alert, moving successful traps regularly in order to confound the rat's formidable survival-instinct memory. Finally, snared animals should be taken to another place to be drowned or have their necks broken: to kill them on the spot might result in 'squealing' which would 'frighten the other rats away'.

A boom in manufacturing followed: each year brought a whole slew of new inventions, innovations in trap design,

poisons promising immediate effect, absolute handling
safety. By the end of the 1920s, books such as Alfred Moore
Hogarth's London-published *The Rat: A World Menace* were
carrying substantial sections of advertisements – for 'Zelio'
paste, 'the new method of exterminating rats and voles . . .
approved by the Ministry of Agriculture and Fisheries';
for the 'one-night wonder' toxin Rodine; for the ruthless-
sounding Cyanogas, which to judge from the illustration
knocked rats immediately insensible, tongues lolling stupidly
from the sides of their mouths; for the downright sinister
Lloyd's Rat Exterminator, 'a new discovery embodying the
use of a powerful Eastern Drug, which has a specific action
on the peculiar structure of the rodent'; and powerful
adhesives such as Dak Ratlime, an 'amazingly tenacious
birdlime [which] ensnares the wiliest and holds the strongest
as easily as a sticky flypaper traps flies'.

Hogarth's text further expanded the theme, furnishing
succulent detail on a whole variety of traps and methods of
snaring. Here, he counselled, a certain profligacy was called
for: 'Do not be sparing in the number of traps, as money
spent in traps is a small item compared to the cost of the
damage done by the rats.' The choice was bewildering:
snap traps, jaw traps for use in burrows, any number of
different kinds of cages; but most appealing – no doubt in
part for the anguished end it inflicted – was the 'varnish
trap', honourable forebear of the glue trap so beloved
of modern-day New York exterminators. On to a strip of
eighteen-by-twelve inch cardboard was spread 'lithogra-
pher's varnish of a certain consistency . . . the rats are
practically always found dead in the morning . . . Most die
of suffocation as a consequence of the mouth and nostrils
being closed with the varnish when the rats attempt to

free their limbs.' Yet just occasionally, Hogarth concluded approvingly, the most effective traps were those which evolved by accident, and at the end of the chapter he reprinted in full a letter first published in the London *Daily Mail*, headed 'Floating corks in a pail of water', and signed 'Helpful'. The discovery of this near-flawless device, explained the gleeful correspondent, had taken place in a wholesale grocer's warehouse, where a bucket of water, with a thick layer of corks floating on top, had been left overnight beside a sack of peas. Come Monday morning, the bucket – the surface of which would have appeared a straightforward stepping-stone to the meal beyond – was 'almost full of drowned rats of all sizes'. Thenceforth, the trap was set deliberately; within a week, 'the stores were rid of rats'.

Of all extermination methods, however, the longest-established appear to have been straightforward arsenic poisoning, and the setting-up of basic baited traps. English chroniclers record rats being caught as long ago as 1297, and Chaucer in his 'Pardonere's Tale' became arguably the first poet to include poison in a rhyming couplet:

> And forth he goth, no lenger wold he tary,
> Into the toun unto a Potecary,
> And praied him that he him wolde sell
> Some poison, that he might his ratouns quell.

Yet the fact that Shakespeare's *Romeo and Juliet*, written in 1592, included a reference to a rat catcher did little to induce ordinary people willingly to become exterminators. By the early decades of the twentieth century, and despite the rat's outlaw status now having been incontrovertibly established, bribes were still deemed necessary in order for dead rodents to begin appearing on Health Department doorsteps. Here, though, the level of the payment, according to one rat-destruction textbook, was critical: 'If too low the premium attracts children only; if too high it tempts fraudulent persons to try their cunning.' All of which made it vital for unpaid predators – owls, kestrels, stoats, even weasels – to be given 'the fullest protection . . . They are most valuable allies and destroy large numbers of rats. It is not a sound argument to object, as some do, that a weasel will not attack a full-grown rat – they will kill large numbers of young ones, and young rats are far more dangerous than old ones. If these beasts and birds of prey occasionally help themselves to a young game bird or a rabbit it is not of much consequence; the rats they destroy will do far more damage.'

*

RATS. THEN, AS NOW, rats were feared and reviled: pariah creatures, known to bite babies, to fight blindly when startled, the subject of myth and nightmare. A century on from the discoveries of Yersin and Simond, the rat has become properly recognized as the health hazard it truly is. It has found its level, earned due recognition as mankind's most persistent and unshakeable parasite, a shadow presence to every careless and wanton human activity, a reminder of our own greed and weakness. The tourism industry, of course, would have one believe that the rat only remains a problem in cities where civic pride has no place – sprawling conurbations synonymous with squalor and degradation, such as Calcutta, Bombay, Surat – and yet the tenaciousness of the creature is such that it can contentedly make its home anywhere there are people. In Manhattan – the very quintessence of the modern city – the war against the rat has never been waged with more manpower or zeal, and yet it has never looked closer to being completely lost.

*

ON WEST TWENTY-THIRD and Ninth, nearing midnight on a driving east-wind April night, a tall stooped African-American was shuffling behind what looked like a steel-tube K-Mart trolley rendered three times its original width by bulging black sacks, each filled and clanking with empty Tab and Coke tins. Despite the cold, he was wearing beach sandals, the rubber soles worn thin as cardboard. He wore headphones, and talked over the hiss of his music.

'Round here,' he said, chopping his hands through the air as if leading the crescendo of some imaginary orchestra, 'we get rats big as this,' – and he abruptly ceased his conducting, and measured a space in front of him the length of a domestic cat.

He beckoned: an infinitesimal – and unsettling – one-finger gesture. He indicated a steel grille in the pavement. 'You ain't seen none? They're watching you. They not stupid. They live down there.' From a distant tunnel came the loose rattle of the subway. 'Sewers, too,' he added.

He looked suddenly over his shoulder, as if worried someone was following him. 'They burrow through wire, concrete. They everywhere, and at night I hear them a-scufflin' and a-scrapin'. Sometimes I have to beat them off with my fists.'

He shook his head, tutted. 'There's lots of stuff people will tell you about rats, lots of stuff you won't believe, but let me tell you now, it's all true.'

*

NEW YORK IS HOME to three species of rat: *Rattus rattus*, also known as the black or ship rat; *Rattus norvegicus*, the brown or Norway rat; and *Rattus rattus alexandrinus*, the Alexandrian or roof rat, which is vastly outnumbered by the first two. Of these, none is indigenous. The black rat originated in India and, most historians agree, disembarked on American soil with the first explorers, having spread to Europe along trade routes during the Middle Ages. The brown rat began life still further east, in central Asia, and started its westward migration early in the eighteenth century. It is a formidable athlete: eye-witness reports from 1729 tell of vast hordes swimming the Volga, then shaking themselves down and shouldering their way into the houses of Astrakhan. Once in Western Europe, its advance was rapid: by the time of the US War of Independence, it had penetrated America and is now by far the most numerous, dirtiest and most visible of the US rats.

Rattus rattus is smaller, measuring about seven inches nose to rump, with an extra nine for tail. It has bluish-black fur which appears to rise in one long hackle along its spine. Its ears, at least compared to those of the brown rat, are noticeably large, their shape reminiscent of radar bowls. It is less likely to be aggressive than the brown rat but, as if aware of this, seldom allows itself to be cornered: it can rapidly shin up curtains, slick-painted drain pipes, elevator cables or telephone wires. It is a formidable acrobat, and can gnaw a hole in a ceiling while at the same time gripping tight to an electric wire.

It is hard to speak of these creatures without a good measure of awe, and even those who have spent a lifetime in their pursuit – men one might expect to have become blasé about the threat rats pose – can be heard reverently lowering their voices, attempting jokes about the animal's prowess that only serve to highlight their own respect. Sitting around a conference table in the New York Department of Health, some eight floors above the streets of lower Manhattan, the city's pest control experts competed to outdo each other in extreme rat tales. The creature was the enemy; their vocabulary spoke, as in San Francisco in 1907, of military manoeuvres against a guerrilla force – rodent inspectors were 'exterminators'; rat infestation they dubbed 'total involvement'; a building overrun from basement to roof terrace was judged to be 'totally compromised'.

The most experienced – and most compelling – of the witnesses was Larry Adams, a rat exterminator of some twenty-five years' standing, and currently the city's 'senior supervisor for extermination'. When he spoke of rats it was with a distinct relish: recounting details of rat behaviour made him smile ruefully, and the more impressive the animal's feat of endurance or strength or resistance the more his amusement grew. He had the excited air of a man faced with a worthy adversary, with an enemy who was always just out of range, constantly moving, more than a match for him in both strategy and cunning.

It was the animal's physical capabilities that struck him as most continually astonishing. The Norway rat, he said, was an 'excellent swimmer, good climber. Poor vision, but pretty fair sense of smell. They're adaptable to anywhere that humans can live. They're attracted to the food we eat, to anything that smells good to us. A double cheeseburger,' he said, smiling slow, 'smells just as good to them as it does to us.'

He warmed to his theme. 'Rats can penetrate darn near anything outside of galvanized steel. They can cut through mortar, brick, wood, even concrete.' He paused, put a finger to his front teeth. 'It's their incisors. If they didn't keep gnawing, their two front teeth would carry on growing, curve back under their chin, drill into the brain and kill them.'

He stopped talking, folded his arms, leaned back. His chair creaked ominously. 'I've seen rats all my life, and I can't stand them. No one who has any idea of the number of ways they can affect you will ever get used to them. You ever seen a baby bitten by a rat? Well now, that's a very unsettling thing, to go into a place and see a child that's been bitten, who's got a chunk of his face missing. Maybe the kid's asleep, maybe got a bit of food or milk on his face. Bam! The rat goes for him.'

It wasn't just plague that rats carried, he added, though plague of course was the best known, the most agonizing and by far the most dangerous of all rat diseases. Others included spirochaetal jaundice, rat-bite fever, trichinosis, Brill's disease and tularaemia.

'The reason they're so difficult to control is that they multiply so fast.' His initial good humour had dissipated; in its place was a stiff-necked resolve.

'A female,' he was saying, staring glaze-eyed out of the window now, 'will drop a litter of eight to eleven rats. Give her a couple of months and she'll do the same again.' The consequences of this were astonishing: it had been calculated that a single pair of rats could – given three litters a year, with ten young in each, abundant food, shelter and zero mortality – increase in five years to something over nine hundred and forty billion (940,369,969,152). In New York, the record reproductive rate – achieved by a single captive pair – stood at seven litters in the same number of months.

He believed that it was largely thanks to man that the rat population was currently so healthy: if it wasn't for the overstuffed garbage dumpsters filled with half-eaten Whoppers and pizza crusts 'rats would control their own population by cannibalizing each other. Since there's always more than enough food to go around, this doesn't happen.'

So, all the bold talk of extermination, the use of terminology more at home in Vietnam or Korea, proved after all to be a smokescreen for a more salutary reality: rats would always be with us, and as the human population increased, so would rodent numbers. Most chilling, for Adams, was the knowledge that there existed in the city locations to which people no longer had access, but which rats had made their fiefdom, areas where they would always be safe, unreachable by trap, poison or fire. 'In this very district right here,' he said, rapping heavy knuckles against the table, 'there are buildings with third-level sub-cellars, structures that date back to the Revolutionary War. I've seen the underground maps of the city, and you'd be astonished what's down there. You can betcha that rats have made a pretty sweet home in these places. And we'll never reach them. Not ever.'

*

IN NEW YORK, at the turn of the twenty-first century, rat catching had become a badge of courage, a stamp of manhood. Gil Bloom, who described himself, unprompted, as a 'hero rat catcher' – ran the same company his grandfather had started in 1929. At nine sharp he was standing outside the Queens office of Standard Exterminating Co.

Inc., headed in his pickup for a job that was 'pretty much typical': an overrun warehouse, where the rats had become so brazen they had begun openly foraging for food during daylight. Like most New York exterminators, he spoke of rats with a tone of measured respect. All the way to the job he pointed out factories, front porches, abandoned lots, each of which might have been expressly designed with the rat in mind.

'Look at that,' he said, gesturing with his thumb as the pickup idled at a stoplight. 'Food-packaging plant. Candle factory. Empty lot. Right next door to each other. Rodents love to gnaw on wax. No shortage of food, either. And there,' he added, as he began to head off, 'an overgrown garden. Right next to it, there's rubbish spilling out of a dumpster. See the problem? The moment you clean rats from one place, they just go right ahead and move across the street, where it's just as nice as where they were before.'

He drew the truck to a halt. Ahead was a yard with an open warehouse at the far end. There were heaps of wooden pallets, steel tubing, a dumpster that seemed to glisten in the pale sunlight as if slimed with cooking fat. 'Check that out,' he said, pointing to a high brick wall topped with jags of broken glass. 'I was teaching a class on extermination one time in Manhattan. I was telling the students about all the latest exclusion techniques, and then we looked out the window and saw a whole line of rodents running along the top of a cyclone fence. That's the way it goes.'

In a windowless plyboard office off the main yard the warehouse manager was waiting. He wore a denim shirt stretched tight over his belly and had skin pale and smooth as kneaded dough. The phone was ringing; he ignored it, stood up from the desk.

'We kept the dog food in the lock box out in the warehouse, and the rats got in under the padlock. Don't ask me how. Then the dog got rat fleas, and we had to put him down. That's why we called you guys in. One rat ate so much dogchow he couldn't get out again.' He coughed drily. 'Now they're coming in here, into the office. One of them has grown so large he's the size of my arm. When I'm working late he comes in through the doorway, stands on his hind legs and stares at me. It's like he's daring me to chase him.'

Outside the office again, in the watery April light, Bloom stopped and kneeled down. There was a manhole-sized fissure in the concrete. He looked up again, nodded at the manager. 'That's a broken sewer you got down there.'

Inside the warehouse, out of earshot of the manager, Bloom murmured, 'Open sewer. Rats live in sewers. They come out the hole, find food, start their little colony. Why don't they get the sewer capped?'

He and his deputy were scouting round the darkness now, flashlights held over their heads dagger-style, aimed downwards. There was evidence of rats everywhere: shredded Styrofoam and silver foil; rat droppings the size of toothpaste squirts and the colour of diseased-dog excrement; corners where the dirt floor had been worn into patterns by rat footfall.

'Sometimes,' he went on, 'you get rats coming up out of the toilet bowl. Alive.'

He began setting up bait stations now – sizeable green plastic triangular boxes, with rat-sized entrances at each point. Inside were blocks of poisoned bait: anticoagulant toxins which, once ingested, took twenty-four hours to kill. However, there was a problem here: the dog food, to which the rats had been enjoying such free access, contained coagulant, a blood-clotting agent added in part to protect canines from rat poison. So, for the toxins to be effective, clearly the rats had to be denied their rations of dog food.

He was concentrating hard, poking the flashlight under piles of pallets, behind the slabmetal workbenches into which colossal circular saws were set.

Back in the daylight again, he said, 'The rats in New York, they're pretty healthy.' He waved an arm towards the barrel of dog food inside the warehouse. 'They get a lot to eat.'

He'd decided against using traps for this job, and no glueboards, either, large cardboard slabs painted with glue and protected, until use, by protective peel-off strips. The glue was so strong rats had been known to chew off their own legs trying to escape. Bloom, fearing that glueboards would be rendered useless in the wet, had opted solely for poisoned bait.

On the way back he was pensive, dismissive about the claims of the municipal authorities to be winning the war against the rat. He was not alarmist, merely realistic.

'There was a novel written a few years back,' he said as he drew to a stop outside his building. He killed the engine; his clipboard was on his knee. 'It was a pulp book about plague breaking out in New York City. I guess most folks thought it was ridiculous, that this kind of thing was real unlikely. But I read it, and it didn't seem that crazy to me. It's a "what if?" scenario. It *could* happen.'

*

UNLIKE SAN FRANCISCO – and, in the early years of the twentieth century, Los Angeles, Seattle and New Orleans – New York has been fortunate and vigilant enough never to have had an outbreak of plague. On two occasions, however, the city has come extremely close. The first time was in 1900, at the peak of the third pandemic. Ports across the world were reporting major and sudden inflagrations of plague and, one night, infected rats were discovered on ships in New York harbour. On that occasion, quarantine restrictions were ordered quick enough for the disease never to make it ashore. The second time, however, some forty years later, was an altogether closer call.

On 10 January 1943 a French freighter, the *Wyoming*, carrying a cargo of wine and tobacco, docked from Casablanca. According to the New Yorker writer Joseph Mitchell, who was told this story some time in 1944, the events that unfolded threatened the safety of the city to such a degree that the public health officials who dealt with it kept the affair secret for more than a year. In the end Mitchell managed to glean the details from Dr Robert Olesen, medical director of the city health service's quarantine department.

Olesen began by explaining to Mitchell the method used for inspecting ships engaged in foreign trade: a five-strong boarding party was dispatched, including a sanitary inspector, whose main job was to determine the degree of rat infestation. This involved a thorough search – looking for rat tracks, signs of gnawing, evidence of droppings and nests. Rats, Olesen went on, 'have a smell that is as distinctive as the smell of cats, although not as rank, and an experienced inspector can detect their presence that way'.

If a ship was judged to be infested, fumigation was

ordered. This was an extreme, and often poorly targeted,
procedure: early attempts using hydrocyanic acid resulted
in the death of a number of stowaways. After this, precautionary tear gas was always released before the poison,
and it had, by 1944, become commonplace to see lines of
weeping and spluttering refugees staggering from the
hatches of South American freighters. After about ten hours,
the holds would be opened up and aired and searched for
dead rats. Whatever fleas were combed from their fur were
ground into pulp and injected into guinea pigs, and the
condition of the laboratory animals monitored carefully and
not without a measure of trepidation.

Casablanca, *Wyoming*'s port of origin, was on the 'plague
list' at the start of 1943 and so her crew was examined with
special care. There was no sign of illness. 'Then,' Olesen
said, 'the captain brought out a deratization certificate
stating that the ship had recently been fumigated – in
Casablanca, if I remember correctly – and was free of rats;
looking back, I feel sure the official who signed this certificate had been bribed.' Nonetheless, on the strength of the
certificate, the ship was allowed to dock. A few bags of mail
were unloaded, and then the longshoremen boarded and
were on the point of beginning to discharge her cargo when
one of them noticed some dead rats. It was not until 18
January, over a week after the *Wyoming* had first pulled into
port, and with most of her cargo emptied from her hold,
that the first rats were finally autopsied. A guinea pig was
injected with mashed-up rat fleas. Four days later, it died.

For the next two weeks, a major covert programme of
rat trapping was conducted on and around the Brooklyn,
Manhattan and Staten Island piers. Early in February the
first of these rats were sent for autopsy. Olesen and his

colleagues awaited the report with 'considerable anxiety. It was negative on every rat, and we began to breathe easier.' Trapping continued for the next two and a half months, and not one infected rat was found. By some miracle, and not for the first time, the city had escaped plague.

The ever-present potential, however – and the prospect of unchecked carnage in such a confined and densely packed population – remains a rich source of novelistic melodrama. To pick just one: *Epidemic!*, an obscure and long-forgotten 1961 procedural about a plague outbreak in Manhattan, author one Frank G. Slaughter. 'The chilling account of a great city's battle against the Black Death!' hollers the subtitle. On the cover, a woman stumbles, hand to her forehead; behind her, in the shadows, a man can just be seen scurrying away, shoulders hunched, collar up.

It is a tale of sudden and virulent contagion, hysterical panic, granite-hearted villains and cool but 'brilliant' doctors, of a city suddenly out of control, open to seizure by the most malign criminal forces. It is also – despite being unashamed pulp – unexpectedly gripping, as well as unintentionally comic.

It starts slow and ominous, with a feverish tramp-steamer captain bravely struggling his vessel into New York harbour. As he changes out of his oilskins, the extent of his infection becomes clear. 'His superbly muscled body dripped with perspiration while he fumbled into slacks and a sports shirt.' As he and his shivering crew stagger ashore, they are closely followed by diseased rats, creatures 'not listed on the ship's manifest, but . . . a sinister part of the cargo she had taken in the Cameroons'.

By the end of chapter two, 'the destiny of New York was truly in the balance . . . The pattern of destruction established by *Pasteurella pestis*, erratic as the finger-painting of a demented child, was now virtually complete.' At this point, 'brilliant immunologist' Eric Stow steps manfully into the frame. Faced with a city in sudden and apocalyptic meltdown – 'Apartment dwellers had already snapped on their burglar chains and locked their windows . . . Theatre and movie houses had seen their audiences reduced to a trickle' – his prescription is blunt. Manhattan has to be sealed off, and he addresses his subordinates in a crowded hospital ward, the general before his troops. '*Pasteurella pestis* has established its beach head. We can defeat it within these boundaries. If we hesitate, we'll have two thousand cases tomorrow in Greater New York. The day after, there could be ten thousand in the metropolitan area alone. Don't think I'm romancing. I've seen this bug in action.'

It is exhilarating stuff which – due largely to the liberal use of hyperbole, the stagy dialogue and the inevitable descent into an Ian Fleming-style struggle between white-knight scientists and an underworld bent on global domination – screams 'fantasy!' from every page. Yet all Frank G. Slaughter did was properly research his field. As preposterous as the thriller undoubtedly is – with its cartoon-impassive immunologists, its square-jawed and resolute police chiefs – there is little that one could decry as implausible. Without the Ernst Stavro Blofeld subplot, *Epidemic!* simply draws on what is already established about the nature and effect of plague upon society. This is known: that few diseases are more contagious or feared, that terror triggers flight, that among those who remain, the worst of humanity results – riots, victimization of the infected, the gradual collapse of order. It had happened in London in

1665, across Europe in the 1340s, in Hong Kong in 1894, and in Surat a century later. Why not in New York?

*

FOR HONG KONG, the cataclysm of 1894 – and the intermittent plague outbreaks that continued until the 1930s – triggered a systematic rat-destruction programme that lasted the entire twentieth century. The first and most controversial move was the levelling of Taipingshan, the central Hong Kong district from which plague had first flared. From the start of the epidemic, establishment opinion, happy to have been able to scapegoat an entire cultural enclave, pushed for demolition and, while the argument spiralled into barely concealed racial jousting, a prison-high brick wall was hurriedly constructed as interim containment. The government, increasingly enthusiastic about the idea of erasing not only disease but any memory of the terror of that early summer, began angling forcefully for the whole area to be first torched, then razed. In Kitasato, as it had no doubt hoped, it found a compliant ally. 'If one desires to properly clean the contaminated houses to make them free of plague,' ran his reply to the letter from the colonial surgeon Dr Philip Ayres, 'it is recommended to proceed radically . . . [and] it is best if at least the inner parts of the houses are burned.' Yersin, whose research into the soil of infected houses had suggested no such certain course, stopped way short of Kitasato. Setting entire streets to flame, he said, was overkill: the microbe in the soil was 'no longer virulent'.

Yet destroyed Taipingshan was and today only the street names and precipitous incline remain the same. The memory of plague, however, died harder and that rare Hong Kong commodity, an undeveloped city block, now

squats in the centre of the neighbourhood in the form of
Henry Blake Park, named after the governor who took over
in late 1894 from the benighted Robinson. This unprepos-
sessing rectangle of shorn grass and concrete walkways had
been intended, so a shopkeeper explained, as 'a kind of
lung, to help us breathe', but it seemed now that few ever
used it, that in fact the Chinese of Taipingshan preferred a
claustrophobic proximity, as they had always done, living at
the turn of the twenty-first century in 1950s slab-built concrete tenement flats, balconies festooned with washing and
cooking pots.

Walking this quarter it was not hard to spot rats, lum-
bering out of the gutter before dusk had even fallen, but
shopkeepers, the moment the subject was broached, would
noisily deny their existence. Voices from the buried dark of
television repair shops shouted, 'No rats! No rats here!' Yet,
just across the street, staple-gunned to a telegraph pole, was
a forty-eight-point warning poster: 'Food and Environ-
mental Hygiene Warning – Poisonous Rat Bait is Being Laid
in this Vicinity'. Another counselled, 'A clean environment
prevents rats. Eliminate hiding places for rats. Do not leave
food for rats. Prevent rats from entering your premises.'

Senior Hong Kong health figures told a different story:
the triumph of order over chaos, of modern science over
what had been a continual cycle of pestilence and disease.
Dr Gerald Choa, physician and medical historian – and
one of those Anglicized Hong Kong Chinese, now in his
seventies, whose pronunciation was more regal than even
the Queen's, with its throwaway actuallys and mind yous
and whatnots – remembered how the 1940s, with plague
still a too-recent memory, had seen ferocious clean-up cam-
paigns. Householders, he said, 'were encouraged to catch

rats and dump them in boxes on the street full of carbolic acid'. Every three months, 'tanks of Jeyes Fluid were put in the middle of the street and people were told to dump their furniture, utensils, clothing and whatnot in there for disinfection'.

Until the late 1980s, rat collection in Hong Kong was pursued on a ceaseless and vigorous basis, the most obvious signs of which were the countless 'rat boxes' secured to lamp posts throughout the city. Little more than ten years on, this now seemed a comically quaint custom, though with the clear volume of rats on the island it was also surprising that the practice had ever been halted. Responsibility for collecting the rodents, explained consultant health department pathologist Wai Ping Mak over the telephone – his manner wry, loftily amused – had been in the hands of government technicians, who emptied the boxes and took the rats for autopsy. Rat collection, he confided, had never been the most popular job, and now that the boxes no longer existed only the most committed operatives were to be found waiting with their foetid plastic bags for the morning doors to Bacteriology to be thrown open.

He turned abruptly serious, and one could picture him holding the receiver away from his ear and frowning, as if the very object suddenly caused him displeasure. 'The real worry,' he said, his voice quieter, 'is the border with China. That is hard to police, and refugees might bring rats and disease with them. But try persuading anyone to pick up rats on the border. The soldiers won't do it, no one will do it. It's becoming a practical problem.'

Which is where it would no doubt remain, at least until plague or another rat-borne contagion erupted once more. No one wanted to admit the scale of the rat problem in

Hong Kong, much less be part of a collection or destruction programme, and on at least one occasion the now-defunct scheme of paying premiums for each rat tail delivered had ended in low farce. This story came from Dr Dan Waters, a long-retired colonial service physician and local history enthusiast who doubled as President of the Royal Asiatic Society.

'The thing is,' he said, his voice startlingly loud, 'the Chinese will always find a way to make money.' In another room of his tiny high-rise apartment a Chinese woman – his wife? housekeeper? – was preparing tea. She brought peanut-brittle biscuits and he nodded acknowledgement, his conversation unbroken, volume undiminished.

'Over the years there have been various programmes to curb the rat population,' he went on. 'At one time you could be paid ten cents for every rat tail you brought in. Now, it didn't take long for the Chinese to see that there was money to be made from this, so they started importing rats' tails from Canton.' One could picture convoys of trucks, waved breezily through customs, then the bewilderment on the faces of health department officials as they handed out ever-increasing wads of dollars.

'This,' Waters said, 'went on until they were found out.' He smiled. 'Yes, great entrepreneurs, the Chinese. *Great* entrepreneurs.'

Chapter Twenty-Two

THE YOUNG DOCTOR was preparing to treat a patient when the bomb exploded. Some twenty years later, he recalled colour, flame, a world hellishly inverted.

'The sky was dark as pitch, covered with dense clouds of smoke; under that blackness, over the earth, hung a yellow-brown fog. Gradually the veiled ground became visible, and the view beyond rooted me to the spot with horror. All the buildings I could see were on fire . . . Electricity poles were wrapped in flame like so many pieces of kindling. Trees on the nearby hills were smoking, as were the leaves of sweet potatoes in the fields. To say that everything burned is not enough. The sky was dark, the ground was scarlet, and in between hung clouds of yellowish smoke. Three kinds of colour – black, yellow and scarlet – loomed ominously over the people, who ran about like so many ants seeking to escape . . . It seemed like the end of the world.'

Nagasaki, August 1945. Survivors, the doctor continued, somehow found their way to his surgery. 'Half naked or stark naked, they walked with strange, slow steps, groaning from deep inside themselves as if they had travelled from the depths of hell. They looked whitish; their faces were like masks. I felt as if I were dreaming, watching pallid

ghosts processing slowly in one direction – as in a dream
I had once in my childhood.'

It was into this scene – already on the scavenge, crawling
red-eyed from sewers and culverts – that the rat slowly and
deliberately advanced. It has become folklore that, after
the obliteration of Hiroshima and Nagasaki, only the rats,
among all mammals, continued to thrive. More likely they
were protected from the blast by being hidden away
underground; in the aftermath, as the earth cooled, great
packs would have coursed down the abandoned, ashen
thoroughfares now bordered by the skeletons of buildings
and the burned spikes of trees, everything still smoking, still
dangerous.

Radiation hits humans and rats – mammals both – with
equal ferocity, but in the Japanese city-targets it was the
people, in daylight, going to work or waiting outside shops,
that were fastest destroyed, their skin melting from their
bones from the heat of the blast and the extreme gamma
and neutron exposure. Rats, emerging later, would have
suffered from fallout, but not before they had feasted on
the ruptured corn silos, the wheat flour still spilling from
bakers' store rooms. When they died, to the collapsed cities'
lists of post-attack perils would have been added the worst:
the threat of plague.

For Cold War scientists, commissioned by fearful
governments to research the effects of nuclear war upon the
cityscape and its population, it was contagious disease that
loomed largest in the catalogue of aftermath catastrophe.
According to the 1987 World Health Organisation report
'Effects of Nuclear War on Health and Health Services':
'Infection would emerge as a major problem. It is a leading
cause of death in victims of burns as well as of radiation.

The epidemiological pattern of disease would be altered drastically in the aftermath of a nuclear war, by impairment of the immune response of the body, by malnutrition, by the lack of sanitation, by the proliferation of insects and microorganisms, which are much more resistant to radiation than human beings, and by the collapse of epidemiological surveillance and disease control. Outbreaks of diarrhoea and respiratory disease would be likely to occur in the surviving population and be intensified by the overcrowding and insanitary conditions of the shelters in which people would have taken refuge.' In the event of 'all-out nuclear war' – a scenario that, in the mid-1980s, seemed far from implausible – 'millions of putrefying human and animal corpses and mounds of untreated waste and sewage would provide a perfect breeding-ground for flies and other insects that are more resistant to radiation than human beings. The uncontrolled growth of insect populations would favour an increase in the numbers of insect vectors of disease.'

Chief among which, of course, was the rat flea, *Xenopsylla cheopis*, bearer of plague, and it was to gauge the likely severity of this disease in the event of nuclear attack that, in 1966, the US Atomic Energy Commission published an exhaustive report. 'Even now,' wrote the authors in conclusion, 'there is only a thin protective wall which guards the human population against [plague]. As the record shows, the wall has been breached occasionally in very recent years ... The universal hardship that might have to be endured with the debilitating effects of radiation exposure and other injuries are very likely both to hasten the conversion of bubonic to pneumonic plague and to increase measurably the chances for an explosive epidemic.'

Plague squats on our doorstep, no longer a disease of

the Far or even Near East, no longer other but very much
here. In the United States, the plague bacillus has been
found in some thirty-eight wild rodents, rabbits and their
fleas; it is endemic among wild rats in the eleven western-
most states; in 1981, a typical year, thirteen people were
infected, four of whom died. A nuclear attack, according to
W. H. Freeman in *Last Aid*, a 1982 investigation into the
medical implications of nuclear war, 'would create almost
ideal conditions for breaching the thin protective wall
against plague. Large areas of the western United States
now relatively devoid of inhabitants might receive an influx
of refugees from threatened or devastated urban areas
. . . Millions of urban refugees, unable to obtain shelter in
existing dwellings, would build earth-covered "expedient"
shelters in undeveloped areas. Such shelters might provide
good fallout protection, but they would create ideal conditions for transmission of plague from rodents.'

In the weeks following a nuclear attack, plague would
dig in, establish itself, become an intimate part of the landscape. As radiation subsided in levelled cities, survivors –
reduced now to little more than rodents themselves, scav-
enging through the wreckage for food, possessions, traces
of lost family – would return to the streets that had once
been their home. Most likely they'd discover only a shell,
artefacts melted beyond recognition: ninety per cent of
housing would be destroyed in a nuclear attack. The only
certainty is that they would encounter disease in unexpected
and medieval forms, of which the most distressing and
manifest would certainly be plague, and, like the most
malign parasite, plague bites harder the worse the circum-
stances. 'Under post-attack conditions,' Freeman concludes
coolly, 'radiation and stress would raise the conversion rate

of bubonic to pneumonic plague to twenty-five per cent.'
With no drugs available and most hospitals destroyed, death
would come quick and pitiless to the surviving homeless,
huddled in the few remaining roofed buildings, black rain
falling all around.

Epilogue

IN THE FIRST WEEK OF September 1894, Dr James Lowson – loyal champion of Professor Shibasaburo Kitasato, and equally painstaking enemy to the best scientific endeavours of Dr Alexandre Yersin – travelled to Japan as honoured guest of the imperial government. He received a tumultuous welcome. A note in his diary, added some time later, reads, 'In Japan . . . was made a national "hero". Valuable presents numerous, and suite of rooms at the Imperial Hotel.' He was receiving his due, proper payment for his role as star-maker.

The visit was also proof, in the world's eyes, of Kitasato's status as sole plague pioneer. It was not the end of the matter, however, for over the coming decades Kitasato's claim to have discovered the cause of plague began to look increasingly shaky and, though he never publicly set the record straight, he too in time would come to realize that his findings were crucially flawed, the victim of hurried research and a precipitate rush for publication. Now, more than a century after the two men faced each other over their microscopes in Hong Kong, the plague bacterium is officially classed *Yersinia pestis*. Yet for most of this time, and certainly during the lives of the two rivals, it was Kitasato who enjoyed the glory.

The conventional narratives – that either Kitasato and

Yersin simultaneously discovered the bacillus, or that Kitasato, as he would always publicly maintain, beat Yersin to
the goal – have been particularly resilient. Such models
of careful scholarship as William Bulloch's 1938 *History of
Bacteriology* state that 'in 1894 Kitasato and Yersin discovered
the plague bacillus', while the alternative line has been
propounded in books like Richard Shyrock's 1947 *History of
Modern Medicine*, which saluted Kitasato as having 'added to
his fame in 1894, when he discovered the cause of bubonic
plague during an epidemic at Hong Kong, and thus exposed
one of the historic enemies of man'.

Returning from Hong Kong, Kitasato lost no time in
declaring that he had discovered the 'virus' of the disease,
an announcement which was faithfully and prominently
relayed in the medical press: according to one journal, the
'people of Nagasaki sent a gold cup to Dr Kitasato for
the honour of his discovery of the pest-bacilli'. In his publications, Kitasato was no less forthright, and seldom passed
up an opportunity to highlight the differences between his
and Yersin's observations, most obvious of which was the
fact that Yersin's bacillus did not react to Gram-staining,
while his coloured easily: evidence of a markedly more
permeable cell-wall structure. Science, he concluded,
needed to come to a 'definite conclusion' as to which of
the two bacilli was the plague pathogen: only then could
therapy and prophylaxis 'be initiated on a truly rational
basis'.

Yet as the old century drew to its close, Kitasato's claim
began to be eroded not by allies of Yersin – as he might
have anticipated – but by his own contemporaries in Japan.
The first stone was thrown by Masanori Ogata, who in 1896
published a paper describing plague research in Formosa

during which he had managed to isolate a bacillus identical to that of Yersin's from infected humans, rats and rat fleas. Any suggestion, he concluded, that the bacillus of Yersin and Kitasato were identical was plain wrong: 'They are two quite different kinds of bacteria.' And it was Yersin's, not that of Kitasato, that caused plague.

By the last months of 1899, Kitasato must have known that his claim was untenable and yet he persisted not only in doing his best to shore up his own earlier shaky research, but in seizing upon every opportunity to rubbish the work of his rival. That year the Japanese government sent Kitasato and three other researchers to investigate outbreaks of plague in Kobe and Osaka and the subsequent report, with its numerous references to plague bacilli, surely ranks as one of the great masterpieces of omission. Nowhere, despite the work of Simond in Bombay, did he mention rat fleas, nor hint at any point that there had ever been any disagreement over the identity of the plague bacillus. The only reference to Yersin was a brusque put-down, a dismissal of his anti-plague serum as therapeutically and prophylactically useless.

There seems no charitable way to read Kitasato's actions: the unavoidable conclusion is that he was step by step trying to erase his previous error in order to protect his reputation. With each publication, his position subtly changed. In 1900, *A Textbook on Plague* by Kitasato's assistant Tohiu Ishigama – a member of the Hong Kong team – stated that there were differences in the bacilli found in the blood and buboes of plague patients. The book – 'revised' by Kitasato, Ishigama's 'revered teacher' – came down heavily and unsurprisingly in favour of the blood-bacillus. 'Professor Kitasato was of the opinion that those [bacilli]

which existed in the glands and other organs were pleomor-
phic involution forms and . . . attached greater importance
to those existing in the blood.'

This convoluted slice of scientific jargon was evidence
of Kitasato further shifting his ground: previously, he had
asserted that the bacillus found in the plague swellings
'was an entirely different species to that which exists in the
blood'. Now, six years after his initial research, his own
bacillus had undergone a remarkable and most unscientific
metamorphosis, to become an 'involution form' of Yersin's
bacterium which first 'invades the blood' as such and
then 'assumes, as it were, a second nature during the septi-
caemic stage of the disease'. This magnificent piece of
fudging enabled Kitasato to surrender to the weight of evidence now supporting Yersin's discovery without having to
admit the errors in his own findings.

When Kitasato died in 1931, his reputation – as he
would have hoped – was safe. Every obituary acclaimed
him as the hero who had uncovered one of science's greatest
secrets, the cause of plague. Only once did he admit his
error, that the bacillus he had found was not the one that
caused plague – and this in private, during plague investigations in Japan in 1899 which unfolded increasing evidence
discrediting his earlier descriptions. In public, in the words
of Norman Howard-Jones's intricately argued 1973 retrospective article in the US journal *Perspectives in Biology and
Medicine*, for the rest of his life Kitasato 'tacitly shared with
Yersin paternity for *Pasteurella pestis*'. To have admitted his
mistake would not only have been a crushing loss of face –
a humiliation particularly grievous for a Japanese scientist
– but would most likely have spelt the end of his dream
of winning backing for a private research institute. So he

dodged the issue, kept his head low, and did nothing to discourage those who persisted in proclaiming him the plague pioneer.

However, there is another player in this, whose shadow in Hong Kong cast such a pall over the work of Yersin, and whose influence was critical in Kitasato's acceptance as discoverer of the plague bacillus. This figure was James Lowson, for whom there was no question which scientist deserved his loyalty: Kitasato was celebrated and venerated – hailed in the press as 'perhaps the greatest bacteriologist in the world' – while Yersin, at least outside France, was unknown. When on 4 August the *Lancet* broke the news that 'Dr Kitasato has discovered and described a specific plague bacillus', it was Lowson who had acted as delivery boy by telegraphing the journal, and no doubt he was the source of the paper's extraordinary coda that 'there will probably be many local *savants* keen on discovering a specific bacillus, and it is necessary to caution against accepting all the statements which will no doubt be put forward in this respect.'

Lowson followed up this first telegraph by rushing a selection of Kitasato's slides to London, which were reproduced in the *Lancet* on 11 August and in the equally prestigious *British Medical Journal* a week later. That day, however, both journals carried a news item about Yersin's letter to the French Académie de Sciences claiming discovery of '*the* bacillus of the Chinese plague'. Yet this was dismissed by the *Lancet*, which cited Kitasato's famed caution and accuracy.

It seemed that Kitasato had rushed into print without having thoroughly tested his assertions. His announcement may have come a good six days before Yersin's, but his descriptions lacked the same forensic precision and, crucially, were unable to confirm how the bacillus reacted to the alkaline Gram stain. His subsequent reports were contradictory and confusing; all signs pointed to a headlong rush to publication, which – though Kitasato had other failings – had never until now been characteristic.

Which leaves just Lowson, the wild card, whose friendship with Kitasato was from the start unreserved and headstrong, his admiration unbounded. Not only did he contribute some of his own slides to the package mailed to London, but the choice of first outlet must also have been his: Kitasato had never published in the *Lancet* before, and would never do so again.

For the rest of his life, Lowson remained convinced that he had backed the right man. Never one to favour diplomacy over brute honesty, he would – at a meeting of London's Epidemiological Society in 1896 – declare with explosive bombast that 'all' Yersin's work was 'suspicious', and that both he and Kitasato had 'little faith in Yersin's serum treatment'. For Lowson, the determination to see proper recognition for his hero – and not for the 31-year-old upstart Frenchman – overrode all proper caution.

Two years before his death in 1935, now back in Forfar, the granite-austere northeast Scottish town of his birth, Lowson took up his 1894 diary one last time. With an unsteady hand, he set about making the annotations that he knew would be read by future historians; the final editorial touches that would, he hoped, leave no room for doubt. By now, he would have realized that Kitasato's claim was untenable and yet he – like his recently dead hero – had gone too far to back down. With hefty pen strokes he underscored what he considered the vital dates and movements – 'Kitasato discovered bacillus' from 14 June, the next day's 'wired *Lancet*' and, under 10 July, 'Kitasato's paper – transmitted to *Lancet*'. At the very end of the diary is a page smaller than the rest, a once-loose notepad leaf, now pasted into the inside of the back cover. Here he repeated the dates, adding 'Yersin found bacillus on 23 June', before concluding with spite and untruth, 'He would not work in the same building as Kitasato and it took him some time to get up a mat-shed.'

*

MOHANLAL STAYED A WEEK, and each day was harder than the last. He had started compliant, offering Hetal a choice – either to return to Surat, or to stay in her parents' village – and promising that whatever she decided he'd stick with her. Secretly, though, he'd hoped that emollience might soften her to his will, for he could not imagine life in such a dusty backwater, could not see how he could survive such boredom and hardship, even with his beloved wife and daughter.

So he returned to the city, and knew the moment he'd done so that he'd taken the right course. The authorities were already setting about a vigorous campaign of demolition and street-cleansing, instituting fines for anyone spotted jettisoning their garbage except in proper bins. It felt like hope, and he wrote Hetal to tell her of his excitement at being part of it. Come, he told her: it is not only I who needs you, but the city also; your city.

He received no reply, and it was another month before his editor allowed him the week he needed to make the trip north and back again. Shorn of his duties as husband and father in those few weeks back in Surat, he'd rediscovered

an earlier self: he'd worked late most nights, part of the
team of reporters now permanently assigned to plague. He,
though, had thrown his net wider than had his colleagues:
where they spent their days tailing the new municipal commissioner, he'd felt drawn to the wider investigation, the
threat of resurgent plague to a world which had for decades
assumed the disease was of only historical interest.

In London, he learnt, a duo of scientists was working
on a greater understanding. From a former colleague,
now on the staff of the London *Independent* newspaper, he
gleaned more: names, research details. Dr Mike Prentice,
Senior Lecturer in Medical Microbiology at St Bartholomew's Hospital, was aiming to demonstrate how the disease
had changed over time and how it might alter in future. Dr
Brendan Wren, Professor of Pathogenicity at the London
School of Tropical Medicine and Hygiene, was looking to
the imminent completion of the DNA sequence of *Yersinia
pestis* as a way of isolating those sections of the bacillus that
were subject to change and which, in turn, could be targets
for new vaccines or antibiotics. Plague, Wren claimed, was
'down but not out'. Prentice went further: 'Given the resur-
rection of whatever conditions allowed plague to spread in
the first three pandemics, there's always the potential that
it could come back.'

As a journalist, Mohanlal was intrigued by these comments, and they proved the starting-point for a series of
front-page stories about the global threat of plague which
thrilled his editor and provided a much-needed circulation
fillip. As a man with his wife and daughter still in hiding,
however, he knew the articles would do little to encourage
his family's return and so, as he arrived in the village once
more, he reminded himself again to accentuate the positive.

Hetal was cooking when he looked in through the open door. Another woman, of about the same age, was holding his daughter. Hetal was talking and laughing, wagging a finger in the air as she reached the climax of her story. Then she glanced up, at the darkened figure in the doorway, and fell silent.

'Mohanlal,' she said quietly.

'You're looking well,' he answered. He nodded greeting to the other woman and entered the house. When he bent to kiss Hetal she turned her head and offered her cheek. It was not until late evening that he was able to be alone with her.

Walking outside, the warmth of the earth rising into the cool black night, she put her arm in his. She talked, and it was immediately clear to him which way this was going. She'd forgotten the simple pleasures of rural life, she said: the focus on crops and animals and the preparation of food. She'd rediscovered a friend from childhood, too, who had a baby the same age. She looked up at him, expectant.

'And Surat?' he said eventually. 'You've asked me nothing about Surat, or our home.'

She did not reply. Away from the dim lights of the village, the black of night was absolute and he could not read her face. He stopped walking, and spoke out loudly till she too stopped and turned and came close to him.

'We're rebuilding the city,' he said. 'Plague was the lowest point, but things are getting better.'

'I love you, Mohanlal,' she replied, taking his arm again, 'but what I saw then scared me. For the moment, I feel safest here.'

So he returned to Surat alone. Six months passed. He saw Hetal once every six weeks, sometimes less, and could sense estrangement growing. At times, she seemed close to surrender, to swallowing her fears and coming back with him. At others, her resolve felt stronger than ever.

His daughter stopped recognizing him, began crying when he reached out to hold her. Most days, as he worked on yet another investigation into the disease that had split his family, he found himself drifting into reverie, imagining that he'd one day look up from his desk to find them standing at the door, that he'd suddenly possess the power to rewrite the past. He knew where he'd start: with that one-thirty a.m. phone call. With that gone they could start over. And on this new morning they'd wake up late and in each other's arms, their baby sleeping still, sunlight streaming through the windows. A day just like any other, simple and perfect and full of possibility.

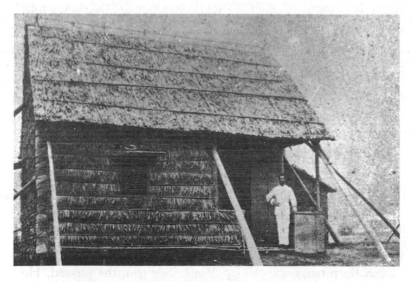

'Dr Yersin at the door of his paillotte', Hong Kong, 1894

Acknowledgements

The research for *The Plague Race* was complex, and I owe grateful thanks to a great many for their patience and generosity:

In Britain: G. P. Amick and the students at the University of Bath Foreign Languages Centre who translated Kitasato's writings from the Japanese for me; Simon Andreae; Will Beck for his Hong Kong advice; Jane Bradish-Ellames whose agenting expertise is sadly no longer available; the polymathic Petra and Paddy Cramsie; Bernice Davison at the London *Evening Standard* for her generosity and flexibility; John Dryden; Jane Durham at Okavango Tours and Safaris; Jan Euden; Jake and Keiko Hobson; Dr Douglas Holdstock for his advice on rats and nuclear radiation; Derek Johns; Ben Jones; Hester Marriott; Richard Milner; Dr Mike Prentice from St Bartholomew's; Denise Prior from the Royal Geographical Society as well as the staff of the society's library where much of this book was written; Susanna Scouller; brother-in-arms Jeremy Seal; Becky Senior; Sally Shalam for helping me get to Madagascar and much else besides; Peter Straus; Dr Brendan Wren from the School of Tropical Hygiene and Medicine; the staff of Hay-on-Wye public library; and Pat from Castle Video for her lunch-hour patience. I also owe a very special debt to Patricia de Mesquita for her tireless and good-humoured translation work.

In Japan: Takeshi Sugiyama from the Kitasato University

East Hospital and Ruiko Oiwa from the Kitasato Memorial Museum of the Kitasato Institute.

In Hong Kong: Dr Gerald Choa; Dr Robert Collins; Ringo Ng and the staff of the Hong Kong Museum of Medical Sciences; and Dan Waters.

In Madagascar: Dr Suzanne Chanteau; Lambo Herizo and his 'bus très fort'; Dr Philippe Mauclère; Glenda Puente; and the staff of the library in the Tana Pasteur Institute.

In New York: Gil Bloom from the Standard Exterminating Company; Russell Galen; Riva Hocherman; and Greg Zareck from Metro Pest Control.

In Paris: Elizabeth Carnier, Daniel Demellier, Dominique Dupenne and Denise Ogilvie of the Pasteur Institute, who were always helpful and courteous. During my first visit to the archives I also benefited from the consummate translation skills and wonderful companionship of Camilla Elworthy.

My biggest thanks, however, are for a single comment made by novelist Raj Kamal Jha at the end of an interview I conducted with him for the arts pages of the *Evening Standard*. It was he who started the whole thing off.